Supreme Health & Fitness by Sean Ali!

Presents:

I0478740

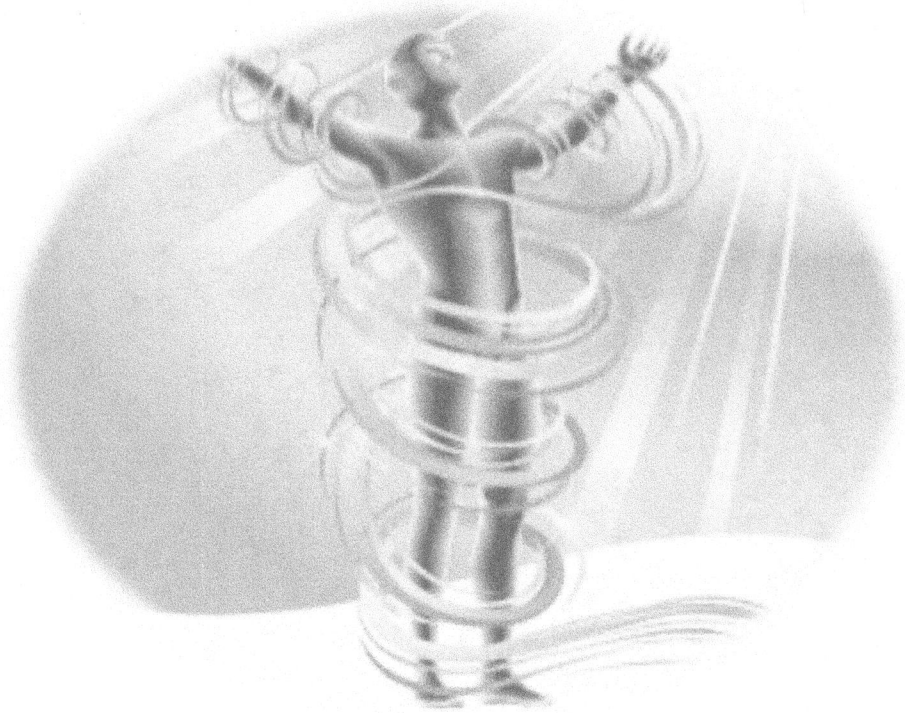

UNDERSTANDING OUR HUMAN ENERGY SYSTEM!

ENERGY CYCLES & TRANSFORMATIONS TO ACHIEVE ABUNDANT LIFE!!

Successfully Building and Maintaining Supreme Health and Fitness by Increasing the level of Knowledge and Science of Life!

Abundant Life Series! * Volume 2

Understanding Our Human Energy System

Energy Cycles & Transformations to Achieve Abundant Life!

******

In our physical world, Energy, like Matter, is neither created nor destroyed. When we speak of Energy being produced, what we really mean is that Energy is being Transformed.

Energy constantly changes form as it moves through various systems. In the human body, metabolic reactions convert the stored chemical energy in food to other forms of energy that carry out body work.

The ultimate source of energy is the sun with its vast reservoir of heat and light. By the process of Photosynthesis, plants use Water and Carbon Dioxide (CO_2) to transform the Sun's Life Energy into Carbohydrates - Chemical Life Energy.

In the body, Carbs are converted to Glucose, which together with fatty acids is metabolized to release energy and support life. The end products of body energy metabolism are water and CO_2. These end products then become available to plants to produce more Carbs or Energy for human use.

Energy Balance is as simple as making better choices and Understanding that our Energy needs should correspond with our level of activity or Energy expended.

Understanding our Human Energy System allows us to make these better Nutritional decisions.

In this book, we explore & examine the dynamics of Energy Metabolism and how to apply for a Healthy & Abundant Life!

Supreme Health and Fitness by Sean Ali!

Achieving and Maintaining Supreme Health and Fitness by increasing the Level of Knowledge and Science of Life!

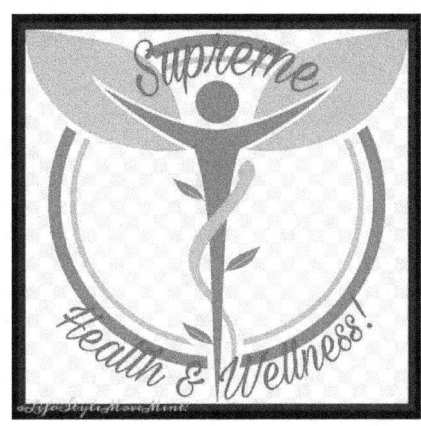

Table Of Contents

****

Page | 7

Introduction

****

Peace and Blessings of Life!

This small book is being submitted so that we can explore and gain an Understanding of what our Human Energy System, while simultaneously being able to properly Apply it to successfully Grow and LIVE to our fullest GOD-Given potential of a Long and Abundant LIFE !!!!!!!

- Do YOU Have health ailments/issues that YOU would like to over-come??

- Do YOU want to Improve the Quality of YOUR Life??

- Do YOU want to Experience and Enjoy ABUNDANT LIFE??

Understanding our Human Energy is synonymous with Understanding our LIFE ENERGY.....it's what keeps us Alive and the main difference between Us and a body in the grave - Human Energy !!!!

Our Energy, and the amount we have, determines and dictates our Health and Wellness. Just as a state of Hunger determines and dictates our emotional state, our amount of Human Energy is the underlying and determining factor of us being Sick or WELL.

If we take and focus our attention to within our Body, we can become able to sense many Life Movements—Flows, Pulsations, Vibrations, Expansions and Contractions and the changing balances of Heat and Cold. In particular we Breathe, and we soon become Aware that to cease breathing is threatening to Life. The entering Breath brings Life; and Breath leaving may even signal its End. This is similar with our Human Energy or Life Energy and HOW we need to focus our attention on Understanding Our Human Energy System. The Leaving of our Energy coincides with the Leaving of our Breath = THE END!

The other side is where we Discover ABUNDANT LIFE......and what my intentions are with this book.

We come from the Earth and ALL our Solutions come from the Earth......All we have to do is simply turn back to the Earth and Extract what we NEED.

We are Earth based, dependent of the Life Element of Hydrogen and the Life Energy of the SUN......that which we can't absorb directly from the SUN, or adequately get from drinking Water we have in the manifested form of FOOD!!!!

Food is the basis of adequately and successfully obtaining Human Energy to Heal, Improve and Extend our Lives and Life-Span.

We can only Grow and Develop as our food is Grown and Developed and is a direct correlation as to the Quality and Quantity of available Human Energy in Self = the foundation for our individual Death or LIFE!

EVERYTHING ADVERTISED/OFFERED IS NOT HUMAN FOOD!!!

We are Naturally occurring Energy/Lives, created from the CREATOR of everything in the Universe. The 'food' we choose to eat should be in-tune with the CREATOR and an Act Of Creation = Naturally occurring Energy/Life as we are = **HUMAN FOOD !!**

WE ARE WHAT WE EAT!!

When the CREATOR brought us into Existence, we already had a Bountiful supply of Human Food = The Garden Of Eden !!!

The Source of our Human Energy System is Human Food........This small book is based on the best Holistic, Scientific and Medical data that addresses WHAT Human Food IS and IS NOT, so that we can make intelligent decisions and UNDESTAND that everything we put into our mouth is either Death or LIFE!

Life Begets LIFE!

Our Lives is Energy based ....Human Energy is derived from the SUN ......manifested IN Human Foods = Fruits and Veggies!!

Unfortunately, many of us don't know How to Eat, what Human food is, our Body parts, number of Bones, Muscles or basic anatomical physiology UNTIL we get sick.....So, with our Knowledge Of Self Series, we aim to introduce You to Yourself!!!

Being educated in the Medical Science field of Health and Wellness added to my qualifications of offering Natural Healing services. Usually someone in my position would put you Back Together AFTER a 'Doctor' practiced an evasive procedure on you, all in the name of Medicine.......**BUT NOT HEALING!**

After witnessing so much damage being done, I decided to take a Pro-Active step and offer and apply my expertise **BEFORE** the body is destroyed. Our Bodies are a Whole and Complete system, with each Organ/System almost intricately connected with each other. Modern medical PRACTICE is based on Surgery/Removal and Medication/Prescriptions. Surgery can be corrective in limited cases, but once a part of ourselves are removed, there is a permanent (often irreparable) disruptions in our Life Energy.

THAT IS NOT HEALING!!!!

THE SAME DOCTORS SEND THE PATIENT TO ME FOR HEALING!!!!

Almost all of the diseases that we seek medical attention for is FOOD/DRINK related. Therefore, ANY procedure, service or program that DOESN'T address this aspect is Only MASKING the root issue and may be potentially causing further harm. In most cases, the procedure is a success but the root issue continues to exist and cause pain and suffering.

WHY?   Because unless the underlying CAUSE is remedied = the damaging EFFECT will still manifest.

No matter how good of a medical professional or the amount of research performed, IF YOUR BODY REJECTS THE PERFORMED SERVICE – YOU WILL NOT HEAL !!

WHY?   Because our Bodies are designed to HEAL ITSELF.........under normal/proper operating procedures.

The lack of solid evidence or an accepted mechanistic explanation for the science of what the "Energy" in Energy Medicine presents a fairly large hurdle with acceptance by Western medicine. This lack of acceptance is translated to the patient, both directly and indirectly, which contributes to the total lack of Knowledge of a large part of ourselves and a major contributing factor in the increase of diseases, illnesses, birth defects and pre-mature death.

Although there is no universal agreement as to what is meant by the "Energy" in energy medicine—or even what kind it might be—terms such as "subtle energy," "qi energy," and prana are often used to describe the same concept or definition of Energy.

Now there does seem to be some consensus on both sides of this discussion that, whatever it is, it is not the Energy currently identified and described by traditional Western physics.

This book represents the Science of *TOTAL BODY HEALING, HEALTH & WELLNES* ....and represents the 2nd Volume of our Knowledge Of Self Series.

Let's Explore and Examine the SAME Science that is used to HEAL your Mind, Body and Spirit AFTER undergoing a Western Medical PRACTICE procedure and see if you can pre-emptively and proactively get yourself to the point where YOU NEVER GET SICK !!!!

PEACE!

Sean Ali, BS Health and Wellness

Supreme Health & Fitness; Owner & Life Coach

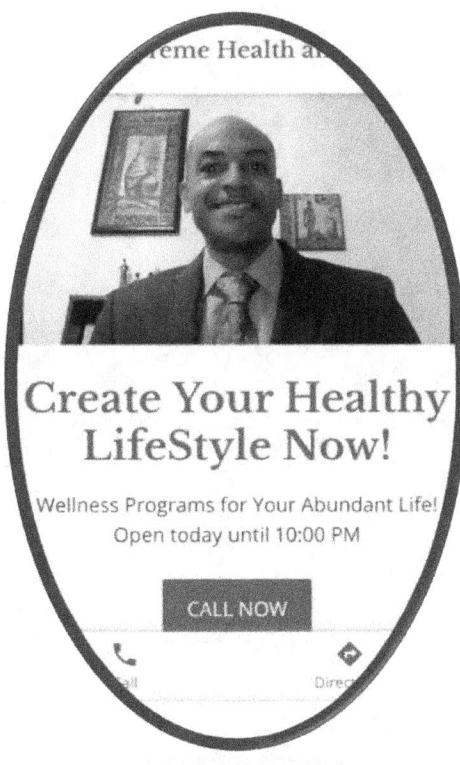

*Chapter One ....

Energy*

******

Everything Is Energy .. Understanding this allows you to Successfully Heal or restore Balance.

Energy is simply the Capacity of a System for doing Work; Energy is manifest in various forms—Motion, Position, Light, Heat, and Sound. Energy cannot be destroyed, but it is Transferred, Converted or Transformed. Energy is interchangeable among these various forms and is constantly being converted, transformed and transferred among them.

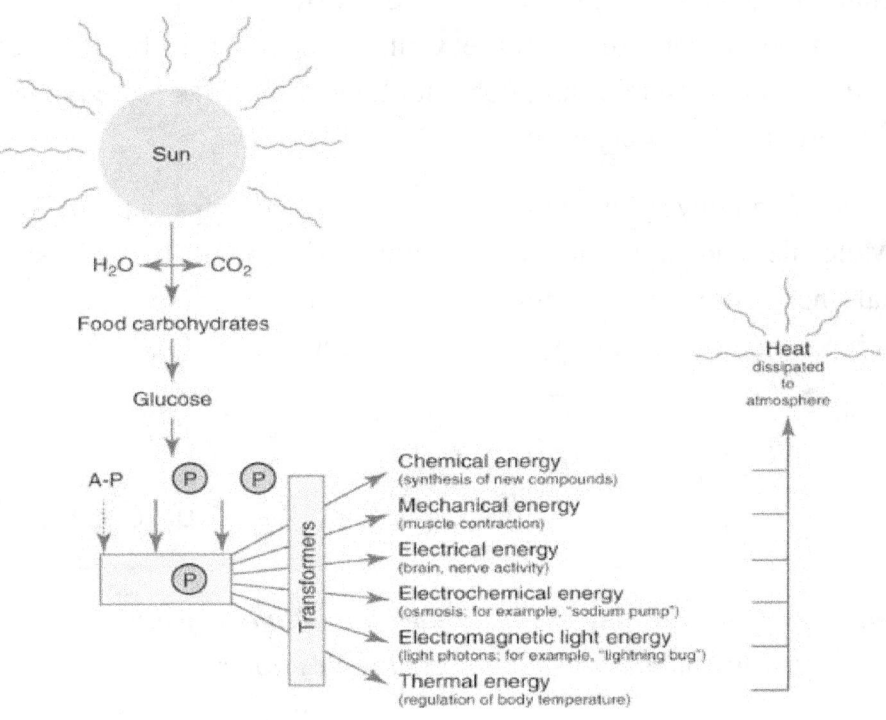

Energy & Energy Medicine

A majority of the Modern definitions for Energy are first introduced to us as grade school students. In the United States, high school students are taught formal (Mathematical) definitions for Energy as part of introductory physics courses. Energy is defined as the Ability to do Work and has two basic forms, Potential and Kinetic.

Potential Energy is essentially Stored Energy (Adipose Fat) and has the ability to do work.

Kinetic energy is literally the movement of things—from air molecules to sound to the splitting of neutrons into atomic nuclei. Kinetic Energy is LIFE ENERGY!

Underlying these deceptively simple descriptions are several subtleties that have been investigated and understood to such an extent that we can harness the Awesome Power of Atomic Energy and with this book we shall examine some of these connections to help us extend and improve the Quality of our Lives = Abundant Life!

Example of Kinetic Energy: the Movement of the needle through the Skin, the Movement of the fluid into the lumen of the vein, and the Movement of the pharmaceutical agent to the Receptor of the Target Cell. Then, in a microburst of activity the Receptor binds the Agent, often releasing Potential Energy that was Stored in the characteristic configuration of the Receptor itself.

The change in Receptor Topology releases the Stored Energy and helps to propel or allow the Movement of Molecules and Atoms across the Cellular Membrane, in the process consuming Potential Energy stored in the Molecule Adenosine Tri-Phosphate (ATP), the universal coin of Life Energy in our Biology of Cellular Reactions and Actions.

Bioenergy source with information content	Transfer medium	Reception and perception

It is at this Energetic Interface that the pharmaceutical industry and much of Allopathic medicine have focused their efforts.

But they are trying to use artificial, manufactured and ma-made elements to prescribe and PRACTICE on us.

CAUSE & EFFECT.........Artificial medicine or substances Cause Artificial Cellular Actions and Re-Actions = the Effect of continued dis-ease and increase in pre-mature death.

We are Naturally occurring Life and ONLY Naturally occurring Life can be of any Help to us or offer any Healing properties.

This previous photo illustrates the space where Endogenous Molecules, as well as pharmaceutical agents, ultimately interact with our Physical selves = Pre-Mature Death or Supreme Health!

These agents Cause and Modulate Cellular Responses through interactions with a class of Bio-Molecules called "Receptors." Sometimes the agent is harvested and acquired from natural sources = Materia Medica.

With modern or Western medicine it is un-naturally synthesized/manufactured in a laboratory, and nearly always it interacts with a Naturally occurring Receptor-type associated with one of our Tissues or organs, or because our Bodies is ONE inter-connected UNIT, groups of our Tissues or Organs.

An un-natural Element inter-acting with a Natural Element might not equate to a Positive Health result. Which just may be the underlying factor as to why we are not living longer despite these 'advancements' in medicine and medical practice.

The point is that all of these steps and the down-stream and side-stream consequences involve the use of Energy (Natural or un-natural) and its Transformation from Potential (Rest or Adipose Fat) into Kinetic (Action or Life Energy) and back again with the additional loss to Heat and randomness at every step.

All Health and Healing therapies utilize and involve these Bio-Chemical, Energy-driven reactions, and thus all Healing is considered a form of Energy Medicine.

- *What is life?*
- *How do we even know that we ourselves are alive, or that others are?*
- *What connects us to the living, and what differentiates the living from the dead?*
- *How much of our world is alive?*
- *Why do some of us appear more vital than others?*
- *Are we born with a certain amount of vitality that we can dissipate and that runs out when we die, or does it fluctuate so that we feel more alive at some times than others?*
- *Are there ways we can enhance our Aliveness or make situations that injure it (such as drug abuse, illness, many childbirths, too much sex, or, as in Chinese Medicine, "taxation fatigue" of qi, the vital energy)?*

Vitalism has been defined as "*the doctrine that the origin and phenomenon of life are due to or produced by a Vital Principle, as distinct from a purely chemical or physical Force*"

To understand Life's enduring Power, it is helpful to consider how we experience being Alive and the ways we think about it, accept and apply it.

Transformation of Energy

When the Stored Chemical Energy of food is taken into our body, it undergoes several changes that Convert it to different storage forms of Chemical Energy. This Chemical Energy is then changed further as Work is performed.

Our bodies use four forms of Energy: (1) **Chemical**, (2) **Electrical**, (3) **Mechanical**, and (4) **Thermal**.

In our Brain, the Chemical Energy is transformed in to Electrical Energy, allowing for the transmitting of Nerve Impulses and the implementing and executing of Brain activities.

Chemical Energy is changed to Mechanical Energy when our Muscles contract; it is changed to Thermal Energy in the regulation of our Body Temperature = **98.6 Degrees**.

This Chemical Energy is also needed for our Bodies to form new Tissues and Molecules for our Growth, Repair, Healing and Metabolism. The by-product of this Work is manifested in the Heat that's given off to the surrounding Atmosphere and larger Bio-Sphere.

In our Human Body, Energy is present as either *Free Energy* or *Potential Energy*. Free Energy is the Energy being used at any given moment in the performance of a task. It is unbound and in motion = *Kinetic* or *LIFE Energy*.

Potential Energy is Energy that is stored or bound in a Chemical Compound and can be converted to Free Energy when needed.

As an example, the Energy stored in a Carbohydrate is classified as Potential Energy. When we eat the Carbohydrate and it is metabolized, Energy is released for our Body to function/work. As Work is completed, this Energy, now transformed/manifested in the form of Heat or Thermal Energy, is given off into the air.

The choices we make for our food directly determines the quality and quantity of Bio-available Life Energy present. This is the catalyst for HOW long we Live and the Quality of our Life-span.

The Measurement of the amount of Heat produced over a period of time makes it possible for us to calculate and express Body Energy consumption in Kilo-calories (KCalories or KCal) = *Units of Heat*.

Energy Balance: Input and Output

A constant supply of Energy is needed to for us sustain the activities Essential to Life, with successfully achieving and maintaining Homeostasis being 1st.

Energy is required to support our internal needs along with the added expectations of physical activity.

Whether this Energy used is Electrical, Mechanical, Thermal, or Chemical, the supply of our Free Energy and the reservoir of Potential Energy decrease as the Metabolic and Physical Work of our body continues; therefore, the system must be constantly refueled from an outside source which we consume through the act of Eating.

For our Human Energy System, this outside Fuel source is Food.

Growing our own food is the ONLY way to ensure that we have the Highest quality, as well as a constant supply of FUEL!

We can only grow and develop as our food is grown and developed…..Growing our own food is literally Growing Ourselves!!

Energy Control in Human Metabolism

If the Energy produced in the body through its many chemical reactions were "exploded" all at once, it would damage our Tissues and Systems, so mechanisms are needed by which Energy release can be controlled to support our Life, not destroy it.

Two means of control make this possible: (1) *Chemical Bonding* and (2) *Controlled Reaction Rates*.

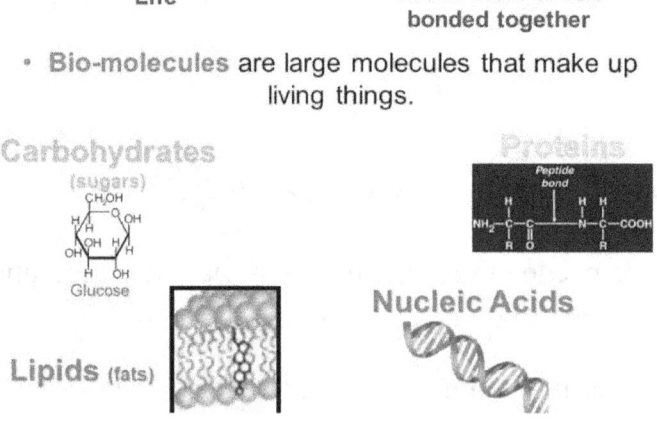

Chemical Bonding

The primary mechanism controlling Energy release in the Human system is Chemical Bonding. The Chemical Bonds that hold elements together in compounds are energy bonds.

As long as the Compound stays intact, the Bio-available Energy is being exerted to maintain it. When the Compound is broken into its parts, this Energy is released and becomes available for Work.

This is a major calculation that we need to include in our Food choices and preparation. The main goal should be Highest Quality Bio-available Life Energy and Maximum Life Energy Extraction.

The following three types of Chemical Bonds that transfer Energy:

1. **_Covalent Bonds_**: These Bonds are based on the relative combining power of the elements that make up a Compound. The Carbon Atoms in Organic Compounds such as Glucose (Life Element) are held together by Covalent Bonds.

2. **_Hydrogen bonds_**: Although weaker than Covalent Bonds, these Hydrogen Bonds are significant because there are large numbers of them. Because they are less strong and more *easily* broken this allows them to transfer Energy easier and more readily from one Substance to another. The Hydrogen attached to the Oxygen Molecule in the Carboxyl group (COOH-) of Amino Acids and Fatty Acids is an example of this type of Bond.

3. **_High-Energy Phosphate Bonds_**: The High-Energy Phosphate Bonds in the compound Adenosine Tri-Phosphate (ATP) are the major Energy source for carrying out our Body Functions. Working like storage batteries for Electrical Energy, these bonds are the controlling force of Energy Metabolism in our Human Cells = *Life Energy*.

Controlled Reaction Rates

The Chemical Reactions making up our Body's Energy System must have controls to manage the speed at which they occur.

For example, some reactions that break down Protein, if left alone, occur very slowly. If such reactions were not accelerated by **Catalysts**, then getting needed Energy from the food in a meal could take years.

At the same time, Chemical Reactions must be prevented from occurring too fast, which would release destructive bursts of Energy.

Enzymes, co-Enzymes, and Hormones regulate Energy reactions as follows:

• ***Enzymes***: Enzymes are Proteins produced in our Cells under the direction of individual Genes. One Gene controls the making of one Enzyme, and thousands of Enzymes exist in every Cell. Each Enzyme acts on one particular substance, called its ***Substrate***.

The Enzyme and its Substrate lock together to produce a new reaction product; however, the Enzyme itself remains unchanged, ready to do its work over and over again (***Figure 1.1***). ***Enzymes often act as Catalysts***.

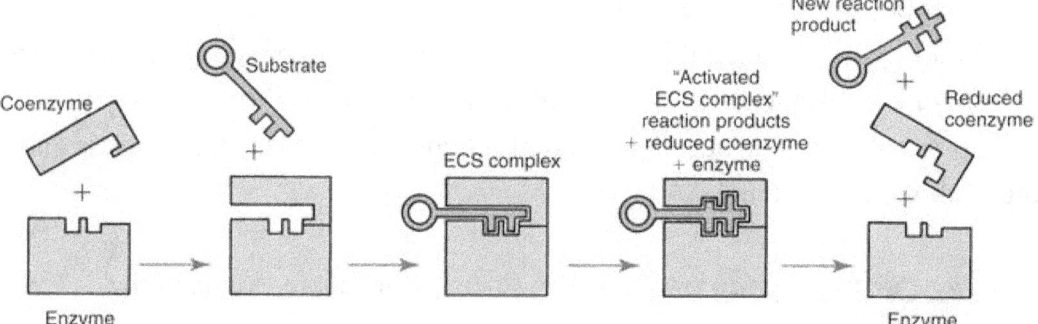

FIGURE 1.1: *Lock-and-key concept. An Enzyme, co-Enzyme, and Substrate work together to produce a new Substance.*

• **_Co-enzymes and Co-factors_**: Many Enzymes require partners to assist in completing their work. These co-enzymes partners are often Vitamins, especially B-Complex Vitamins.

A variety of Minerals also participate in Enzyme reactions and in this role are referred to as **_co-factors_**. It may be helpful to think of co-enzymes and co-factors as another Substrate, because in receiving the material being transferred, they are changed or reduced.

• **_Hormones_**: In Energy Metabolism hormones act as messengers to trigger or control Enzyme action. The rate of Oxidation reactions in the tissues—our Body's Metabolic Rate—is controlled by **_Thyroxine_** (T_4) from our Thyroid Gland. Another example is the controlling action of i\Insulin on Glucose utilization in our Cells.

Types of Metabolic Reactions

Two types of reactions occur in the body: (1) Anabolic and (2) Catabolic. Each of these reactions requires Energy. The process of Anabolism synthesizes new and more Complex Substances as in body growth and repair.

The process of Catabolism breaks down Complex Substances to more simple ones, as when worn-out proteins are broken down and their released Amino Acids used to make new Proteins. Both activities release Free Energy, but the work performed also uses up some Free Energy.

This creates a constant Energy deficit that must be met by food.

Growing our own food and practicing the principle of eating to live is the best way to ensure the consumption of the highest Quality of Life Energy available. This allows us to successful Build and Maintain our own Supreme Health and Fitness!

If we examine the current epidemic of the rise of Obesity and its associated health issues, we can see the close correlation to food choices and the Toxic Energy released when consumed.

Sources of Stored Energy

When a person is not taking in food, as in fasting or starvation, the body must draw on its own stores for energy. Sources of stored energy can meet short- or long-term needs, as described below:

• *__Glycogen__*: there is Only a 12- to 36-hour reserve of Glycogen that can be manifested in our Liver and Muscle; it is *quickly* depleted.

• *__Muscle mass__*: Energy stores in the form of Muscle Protein exist in limited amounts but in greater volume than Glycogen stores. Although the body tries to limit the break-down of Protein for Energy, the need for Glucose to fuel our Central Nervous System (CNS) results in loss of our Body Protein when Energy and Carbohydrate intakes are inadequate. Loss of Body Protein occurs in rapid weight loss and in body wasting or **Cachexia**. It is a cause for concern and requires prompt intervention.

• *__Adipose (Fat) Tissue__*: Even though Fat stores are generally the largest resource of stored Energy, the supply varies from person to person, mainly dependent on the amount of Body Fat available on the individual.

ENERGY SOURCE	KCALORIES PER GRAM
Carbohydrate	4
Protein	4
Fat	9
Alcohol	7

Measurement of Energy Balance

Approximate Composition

An alternative method of estimating the energy value of a food is by calculating the Kcals contributed by the carbohydrate, fat, and protein content as listed in food tables.

These calculations are based on the Kcals value per gram of each of the energy-yielding macronutrients, values known as their *Fuel Factors*.

Note that 1 gram of Fat contains *more than twice* the number of Kcals as 1 gram of Carbs or Proteins. The Fuel factor for Alcohol (7 Kcal/g) falls midway between that of Fat and that of Carbs and protein.

Using the method of approximate composition, a <u>food containing 12 g of Carbes, 8 g of Protein, and 5 g of Fat would contain 125 Kcals</u>.

Kilocalorie

Because the resultant release of Energy and Work performed by our body produces Heat, this Energy Expenditure can be effectively calculated or measured in Heat Equivalents. This measure of heat is the **Calorie**. To avoid having to calculate very large numbers, health professionals use the **Kilocalorie** (Kcals)to describe our Energy needs.

The Kilocalorie is equal to 1000 Calories, which represents the amount of heat required to raise 1 kilo-gram of Water 1° C. (Materials prepared for the general public use the term *calorie*, although the actual measurement is the kilocalorie.)

Joule

The international (*Système International d'Unités* [SI]) unit of Energy measurement is the **Joule**. It equals the Amount of Energy Expended when 1 kilo-gram of a substance is moved 1 meter by a Force of 1 Newton (N). The conversion factor for changing Kcalories to Kilo-Joules (kJ) is 4.184 (1 kcal = 4.184 kJ).

Some nutrition research journals use kilojoules rather than kcalories to describe energy intakes; in clinical practice we use kcalories.

Food Energy Measurement

When striving to help people develop a food pattern appropriate to their Energy needs, it is necessary to know the Energy Content of individual foods. There are two methods for determining the Energy Content of foods: (1) Direct Calorimetry or (2) Calculation of Approximate Composition.

Total Energy Requirement

The Total Energy expended by an individual stems from three Energy needs: (1) ***Basal Metabolism,*** (2) ***Food Intake Effect***, and (3) ***Physical Activity***.

Physical size and Body Composition, as well as the level of physical activity, influence the Energy needs of a given individual. Eating more than required contributes to gaining unnecessary weight as the unused Energy is converted into Adipose Fat Tissue.

Food Intake Effect (Thermic Effect of Food)

Taking in food stimulates our bodies Metabolism because Energy is needed to Digest, Absorb, Metabolize, and Store nutrients. The Kcals needed to perform these tasks is called the **Thermic Effect of Food (TEF)**.

On average, approximately 10% of the kcals in a meal or snack are used to process and metabolize that food, although this varies depending on the meal composition. Foods that are easily digested use less. Proper food combinations utilize less Energy.

Improperly combined meals increase the amount of Energy needed and expended to digest the meal.

Macro-nutrients differ in their TEFs. The TEF for Fat is 0% to 3%, because fatty acids are easily Burned for Energy or Stored in the form in which they enter the body (Adipose Fat); therefore, few Kcalories are needed for processing or storage.

For Carbohydrate the TEF is 5% to 10% of its Kcals.

For Protein the TEF is 20% to 30% of its Kcal content.

The TEF for alcohol is 10% to 30%.

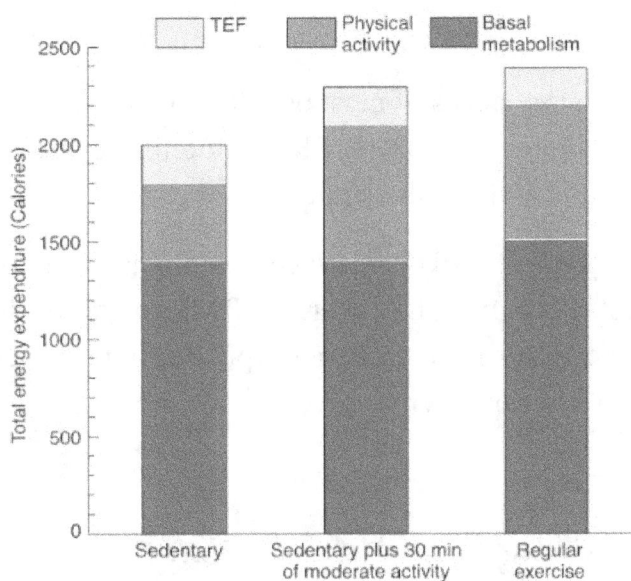

The Energy or Nutrients in food fuel our activity, and physical activity in turn affects our energy and nutrient needs. Both food and physical activity are necessary for optimal health.

The total amount of energy we expend each day is the sum of the energy used for asal Metabolism, physical activity, and the ***Thermic Effect of Food*** (TEF).

Adding 30 minutes of Moderate Activity to a sedentary lifestyle can increase Energy Expenditure by as much as 300 Calories. A program of regular exercise increases muscle mass, which increases basal metabolism, further increasing Total Energy Expenditure.

Basal Metabolic Rate

The **Basal Metabolic Rate (BMR)** is a measure of the Energy required to maintain our bodies during our state of Rest. This is the sum of all the Chemical activities going on in our body plus the Energy needed to fuel our Brain, Heart, Lungs, Kidneys, and other Organs that must continue to work even when the body is in a state of Rest.

Certain small but Active Tissues such as our Brain, Liver, Gastrointestinal Tract, Heart, and Kidneys make up less than 5% of Total body weight but add up to about 60% of Basal Metabolic Activity.

The BMR is the largest of the energy needs of most people, accounting for 60% to 70% of the total daily Energy Expenditure. Thus, the BMR is seldom measured in clinical practice because of the preparation and details required.

Rather, the ***Resting Metabolic Rate*** **(RMR)** is more commonly used because it does not require Fasting prior to the test. Recognize, however, the RMR may be as much as 10% to 20% higher than the BMR because of energy being expended in the processing of food or the delayed effect of recent physical activity.

Measuring Basal Metabolic Rate

The BMR can be measured by Direct or Indirect methods of Calorimetry, as follows:

• ***Direct calorimetry***: Using the direct method, a person is placed in an enclosed chamber that has the capacity to measure body heat production while the person is at rest. This instrument is large and costly and usually found only in research facilities.

• ***Indirect calorimetry***: Using the indirect method, a portable instrument called a *respirometer* is brought to the side of the bed or chair. This complete apparatus is often referred to as the ***Metabolic Cart***. As the person breathes through a mouthpiece or ventilated hood, the exchange of gases in respiration, called the ***Respiratory Quotient*** (CO_2/O_2), is measured.

Because more than 95% of our bodies Energy comes from Oxygen-related reactions and the BMR can be calculated from the amount of Oxygen consumed in a given period. The amount of Oxygen used equals the amount of Heat released. These numbers can be converted to kcals using standardized equations.

• **_Indirect laboratory tests_**: The BMR is regulated by the Thyroid Hormone Thyroxine (T_4); thus Thyroid function tests can provide indirect measures of BMR andTthyroid activity.

These tests include measurements of serum Thyroid-Stimulating Hormone (TSH) from the Anterior Pituitary Gland, as well as Tri-Iodothyronine (T_3) and T_4.

Thyroid Hormone levels within the normal range indicate that Cell metabolism is occurring at normal rates but cannot be used to calculate BMR.

Factors Influencing Basal Metabolic Rate

Individual characteristics including gender, body size and composition, genetic makeup, and disease state influence the BMR of an individual, explained as follows:

• **_Body size and body composition_**: Lean body mass (LBM) is the body compartment made up of muscle and vital organs. It is the major factor influencing BMR because of the high metabolic activity of these tissues compared with the less active tissues of fat and bone. Differences in Basal Energy requirements between men and women of the same height and body weight relate to their differences in body composition. Compared with men, women have less muscle and more fat, resulting in a lower BMR. As humans age, the loss of muscle tissue and to a lesser extent organ tissue, lowers their BMR.

• **_Growth_**: The increased anabolic work supported by growth hormone adds to the BMR in childhood, adolescence, pregnancy, and lactation.

• **_Fever_**: With a fever the BMR increases approximately 7% for each 1°F (0.83°C) rise in body temperature.

• **_Disease_**: Diseases that increase Cell activity such as cancer, cardiac failure, and chronic obstructive pulmonary disease increase BMR and often result in loss of body weight and muscle. Renal disease and Sepsis increase the metabolic work of the body and the BMR. The involuntary muscle tremors of Parkinson's disease increase energy needs. Older adults with pressure ulcers have increased basal requirements, and untreated Human Immunodeficiency Virus (HIV) infection can raise Resting Energy Expenditure (REE) by more than 10%. Standard prediction equations based on height and weight underestimate the BMR of children with cystic fibrosis. Conversely, in starvation and protein-energy malnutrition, BMR falls as cell metabolism slows in response to the drop in energy intake and loss of metabolically active tissue.

• **Climate**: BMR rises in response to lower environmental temperatures as the body takes action to increase heat production and minimize heat loss. Opposite reactions that reduce heat production and increase heat loss as environmental temperatures rise also raise the BMR. Unless weather conditions are extreme, these changes in BMR are temporary while the individual adapts to the new environment.

• **_Genetics_**: Race and ethnicity influence BMR. African Americans have a lower REE per unit of LBM than Caucasians, which may relate to the smaller size of organs with high metabolic rates. Energy prediction equations developed with Caucasian youth do not accurately predict REE in obese Hispanic youth. Studies of the human genome indicate that intrafamily differences in RMR may contribute to higher weight gain and development of metabolic syndrome among particular groups.

• **_Age_**: Loss of LBM, particularly muscle, results in a drop in REE in frail older adults.

ENERGY EXPENDITURE PER POUND PER HOUR FOR VARIOUS ACTIVITIES

ACTIVITY	Kcal/lb/hr*
Daily Activities	
Cleaning	1.36
Cooking	0.91
Driving a car	0.91
Gardening	1.81
Reading, writing while sitting	0.70
Sleeping	0.41
Shoveling snow	2.72
Walking	
Moderate: 3 mph (20 min/mile), level	1.50
Moderate: 3 mph (20 min/mile), uphill	2.73
Brisk: 3.5 mph (17 min/mile), level	1.72
Fast: 4.5 mph (13 min/mile), level	2.86
Running	
5 mph (12 min/mile)	3.63
7 mph (8.5 min/mile)	5.22
9 mph (6.5 min/mile)	6.80
Bicycling	
Light (10-11.9 mph)	2.72
Moderate (12-13.9 mph)	3.63
Fast (14-15.9 mph)	4.54
Sports	
Field hockey	3.63
Golf	2.04
Rollerblading	4.42
Soccer	3.85
Swimming, moderate	3.14
Volleyball	1.81
Weight Training	
Light or moderate	1.36
Heavy or vigorous	2.72

Multiply activity factor by weight in pounds by fraction of hour performing activity. Example: a 150-lb person plays soccer for 45 minutes, as follows: 3.18 (factor) × 150 (lb) × 0.75 (hr) = 357.75 calories burned.

Energy expenditure also depends on an individual's physical fitness and continuity of exercise.

Estimating Energy Requirements

Estimating the total energy requirement for a given individual is difficult. An expert panel defined the *Estimated Energy Requirement* (EER) as the energy intake that will maintain the Energy Balance in a healthy adult of a certain age, gender, weight, height, and level of physical activity, and developed some numerical equivalents to assist in calculation.

FACTORS FOR CALCULATING DAILY ENERGY EXPENDED IN PHYSICAL ACTIVITY

ACTIVITY LEVEL	DEFINITION	PHYSICAL ACTIVITY FACTOR*
Sedentary	Normal activities required for independent living	0.2
Low active	Normal activities required for independent living plus at least 30 to 60 min of moderately intensive activity	0.5
Active	Normal activities required for independent living plus *more* than 60 min of moderately intensive activity or a mix of moderately intensive and vigorous activity	0.7
Very active	Normal activities required for independent living plus 2 hours or more of vigorous activity	1.2

These physical activity factors represent the midpoint of the range for each activity level.

Adapted from Food and Nutrition Board, Institute of Medicine: *Dietary Reference Intakes for energy, carbohydrate, fiber, fat, fatty acids, cholesterol, protein, and amino acids (macronutrients)*, Washington, D.C., 2002, National Academies Press.

Typical ranges for RMR are 0.8 to 1.0 kcal/min for women and 1.1 to 1.3 kcal/min for men (1 kcal/min is about equal to the heat released by a burning candle or 75-watt bulb over the course 180of a minute). Differences in body dimensions and the proportion of body fat versus muscle influence the RMR and thus the total energy requirement. Individuals with a greater amount of body fat and a lesser proportion of muscle will likely need fewer Kcals.

Because your RMR reflects your body weight, your energy expenditure in physical activity can be calculated using a factor that estimates your activity level.

Nutrition experts have defined several levels of physical activity and developed factors that estimate the kcalories required.

 Consider these definitions and the time span and intensity of activity required. If your only physical activity for the day involves the casual walking and routine tasks we all perform as part of our daily living, then your pattern is sedentary.

Additional activity in the form of walking at a brisk pace, running, dancing, sports, or use of fitness equipment is needed for the higher categories of activity. Estimate your personal activity level by keeping a daily record; you may be less active than you think you are.

The Speed at which a person Moves also influences the number of Kcals expended. Walking at a speed of 4 mph requires more Kcals than walking at 2 mph, regardless of body weight. Jogging or running at 5 mph requires *more than twice* the Energy than walking at 3.5 mph.

ESTIMATED ENERGY REQUIREMENTS (EERs) BASED ON ACTIVITY LEVEL AND AGE

	MALE (178 lb, 71 in)* KCALORIES		FEMALE (132 lb, 61 in)* KCALORIES	
ACTIVITY LEVEL	Age 25	AGE 65	AGE 25	AGE 65
Sedentary	2685	2285	1869	1589
Low active	2934	2534	2072	1792
Active	3250	2850	2325	2045
Very active	3770	3370	2628	2348

The Energy cost of Movement is also influenced by age-related changes in Muscle Mass and Innervation of Muscle Cells. Older adults had an energy cost 20% higher than younger adults walking a similar distance at the same speed on a level surface.

The slower gait observed among older individuals may be a compensatory response to offset the greater energy cost of walking brought about by aging and chronic conditions.

New Research Exploring Total Energy Expenditure

As the prevalence of overweight grows worldwide, medical scientists are exploring Physiologic and Metabolic factors that might influence Energy Intake as well as Energy Expenditure.

New areas of research with potential for future intervention include the following:

• ***Action of intestinal microflora***: Particular species of Intestinal Bacteria may have a role in prevention and treatment of obesity.

When the quantities of Fatty Acids produced by bacterial fermentation exceed the amount needed by the Intestinal Cells, the excess are absorbed into the body, adding to Energy Intake. Obese individuals have a different profile of Intestinal Microflora than the non-obese, and introduction of useful microflora might assist in weight management.

• **_Brown fat thermogenesis_**: Brown Fat is a special adipose tissue capable of high energy metabolism given off as Heat. Infants have plentiful amounts of Brown Fat to assist in their response to cold as they move from the warmth of the womb to the ambient temperature surrounding them. Brown Fat is lost as individuals move through childhood and adolescence, although adults retain small amounts. Brown Fat affects long-term Energy balance by raising the BMR. Capsaicin, a compound found in hot peppers, activates Brown Fat thermogenesis in some individuals.

• **_Sleep deprivation_**: It is estimated that 30% of Americans get 6 or fewer hours of sleep per night, as life becomes more demanding.

Too little sleep influences energy intake and expenditure in several ways:

(1) Sleep-deprived individuals often experience increases in appetite and crave snack foods high in carbohydrate and fat;

(2) Lack of sleep reduces one's energy level so that active pursuits are likely avoided; and

(3) Hormonal changes set up metabolic patterns that contribute to body weight gain. Night shifts and rotating work shifts can disrupt body metabolism and promote unwanted weight gain. Increasing hours of sleep may help bring about weight loss or prevent unwanted weight gain.

People who carry their excess fat around and above the waist have more visceral fat. Those who carry their extra fat below the waist, in the hips and thighs, have more subcutaneous fat. In the popular literature, these body types have been dubbed "apples" and "pears," respectively.

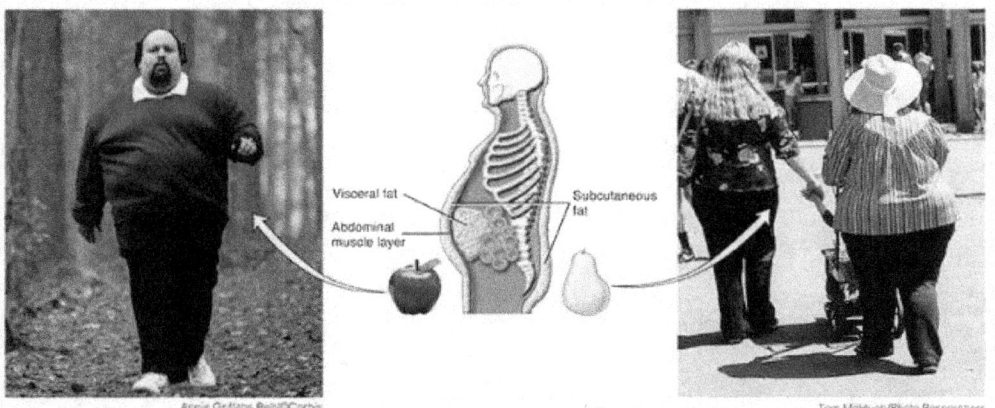

Waist circumference is indicative of the amount of visceral fat, the type of fat that is associated with increased health risk. Waist measurements along with BMI are used to estimate the health risk associated with excess body fat. These waist circumference "cutpoints" are not useful in patients with a BMI of 35 kg/m^2 or greater.

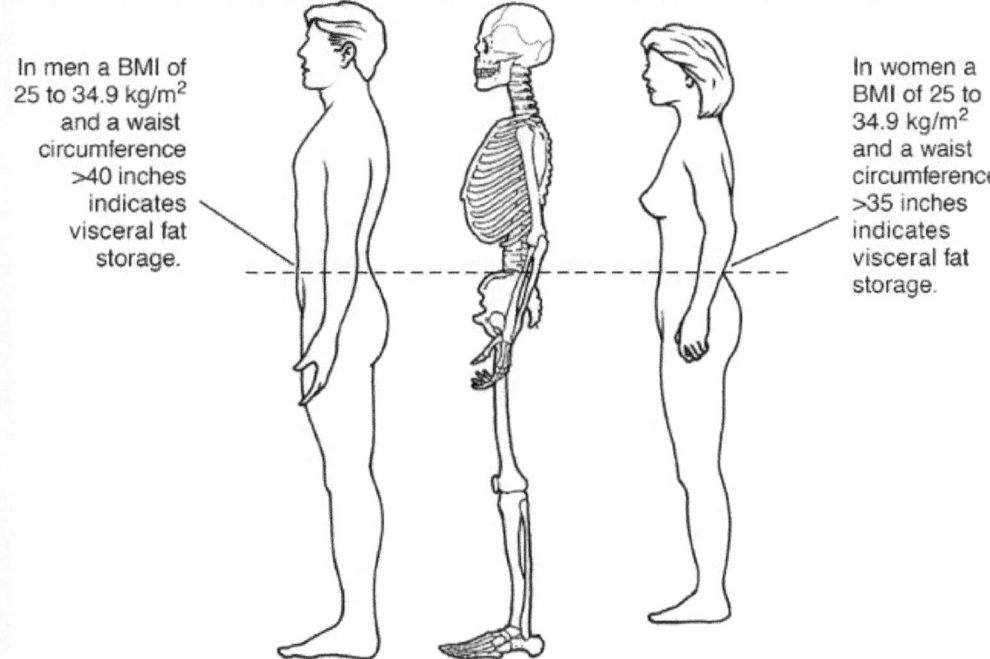

In men a BMI of 25 to 34.9 kg/m^2 and a waist circumference >40 inches indicates visceral fat storage.

In women a BMI of 25 to 34.9 kg/m^2 and a waist circumference >35 inches indicates visceral fat storage.

*Chapter Two ...

Energy Imbalances*

****

The increasingly high rate of overweight and obesity in virtually every population group in the United States demonstrates that many Americans have a dangerous Energy Imbalance. According to the principle of **Energy Balance**, if you consume the *same* amount of—or calories—as you expend, your body weight will remain the *same*.

If you consume *more* Energy than you expend, you will *gain* weight, and if you expend *more* Energy than you consume, you will *lose* weight. For many in the United States today, Energy Intake is exceeding their Energy Expenditure. Bringing it back into balance requires an understanding of how many Kcalories we need and how we use this Energy.

<u>*Energy Balance*</u>- The amount of Energy *Consumed* in the diet compared with the amount *Expended* by the body over a given period.

America's Energy Imbalance

In the United States today, almost 69% of adults are either overweight or obese.[1] Carrying excess body weight usually involves excess body fat, which increases the risk of a host of chronic diseases. The number of people who carry excess fat has increased dramatically over the past five decades. In 1960, only 13.4% of American adults were obese. By 1990, about 23% were obese, and today almost 35% are obese. Excess body weight and fat are a major public health concern that affects both men and women of all ages and all racial and ethnic groups. Obesity rates for minorities often exceed those in the general population: Almost 48% of African Americans and over 42% of Hispanic Americans are obese.

Adipose Fat Tissue is POTENTIAL ENERGY manifested in Atomic form….and is a naturally occurring process that involves Self-Preservation to prevent starvation and maintain our Life through an emergency or extreme measures.

Our Movement 'burns' or uses the Adipose Fat Tissue, converting the Mass into Energy to Move…..Which is the primary reason a Sedentary lifestyle has so many negative health issues associated with it. The more one remains motionless for longer durations = the more Adipose Fat Tissue/Potential Energy collected and unused.

Overweight Being too heavy for one's height, usually due to an excess of body fat. Overweight is defined as having a Body Mass Index (ratio of weight to height squared) of 25 to 29.9 kilograms/ meter^2 (kg/m^2).

Obese Having excess body fat. Obesity is defined as having a Body Mass Index (ratio of weight to height squared) of 30 kg/m^2 or greater.

Over the past several decades, changes in our food supply and lifestyle have affected what we eat, how much we eat, and how much exercise we get. Simply put, more Americans are overweight than ever before because we are eating more and burning fewer calories than we did 40 or 50 years ago.

Food is plentiful and continuously available, and little activity is required in our daily lives.

Being overweight also has significant psychological and social consequences. Overweight and obese individuals of any age are at increased risk of experiencing depression, negative self-image, and feelings of inadequacy.

They may also be discriminated against in college admissions, in the workplace, and even on public transportation. The physical health consequences of excess body fat may not manifest themselves as disease for years, but the psychological and social problems are experienced every day.

Location of Body Fat

The location of body fat stores affects the risks associated with having too much fat . Excess Subcutaneous Fat, which is adipose tissue located under the skin, does not increase health risk as much as does excess Visceral Fat, which is Adipose Tissue located around the organs in the Abdomen.

Generally, Fat in the hips and lower body is Subcutaneous, whereas Fat in the abdominal region is primarily Visceral.

An increase in Visceral Fat is associated with a higher incidence of heart disease, high blood cholesterol, high blood pressure, stroke, type 2 diabetes, and some types of cancer.

Eating more

Today In America we have supermarkets, fast-food restaurants, and convenience marts make palatable, affordable food readily available to the majority of the population 24 hours a day. We are constantly bombarded with cues to eat: Advertisements entice us with tasty, inexpensive foods, and convenience stores, food courts, and vending machines tempt us with the sights and smells of fatty, sweet, high-calorie snacks.

As a result, since 1970 the amount of energy available to us has increased by about 600 Calories per day, with the greatest increases in added fats, grains, dairy products, and sweeteners. The accessibility of tempting treats stimulates the **Appetite**.

Because Appetite is triggered by external cues such as the sight or smell of food, it is usually Appetite, and NOT **Hunger**, that makes us stop for an ice cream cone on a summer afternoon or give in to the smell of freshly baked chocolate chip cookies while strolling through the mall. Studies examining the relationship between the food environment and BMI have found that people in communities with more fast-food or quick-service restaurants tend to have higher BMIs.

Appetite- A desire to consume specific foods that is independent of hunger.

Hunger- A desire to consume food that is triggered by internal physiological signals.

In addition to having more enticing choices available to us, we consume more calories today because portion sizes have increased (*Figure Below*). The more food that is put in front of people, the more they eat. Portion size is associated with body weight; being served and consuming larger portions is associated with weight gain, whereas small portions are associated with weight loss.

Portion Distortion

The burger and French fry portions served in fast-food restaurants today are two to five times larger than they were when fast food first appeared about 50 years ago.

Soft-drink portion sizes have also escalated. A large fast-food soft drink today contains 32 ounces, providing about 300 Calories, and 20-oz bottles have replaced 12-oz cans in many vending machines.

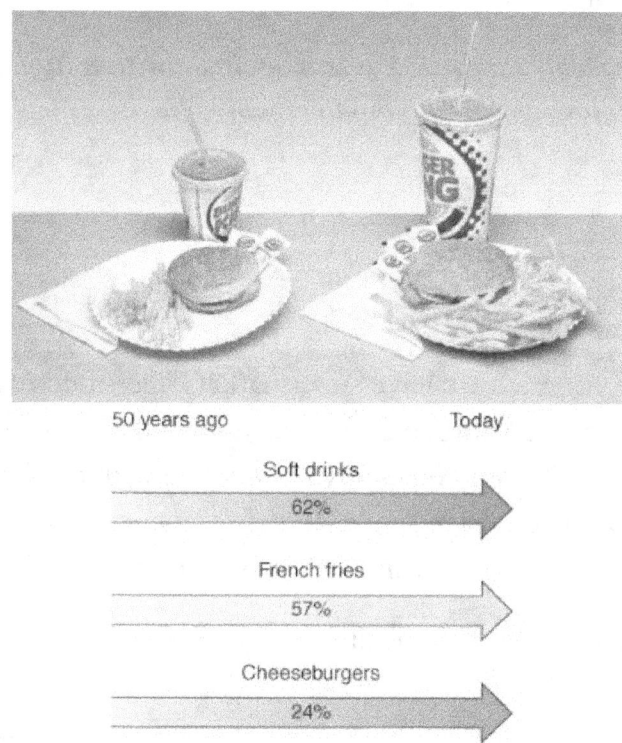

50 years ago   Today

Soft drinks
62%

French fries
57%

Cheeseburgers
24%

Percentage increase in portion size

Social changes over the past few decades have also contributed to the increase in the number of calories Americans consume. Busy schedules and an increase in the number of single-parent households and households with two working parents mean that families are often too rushed to cook meals at home. In conclusion, these prepackaged, convenience, and fast-food meals have become mainstays. *These foods are typically higher in Saturated Fat and Low-density and Toxic Energy than foods prepared at home*.

Moving less

Along with America's rising low-density and toxic energy intake, there has been a decline in the amount of energy Americans expend, both at work and at play. Fewer American adults today work in jobs that require physical labor.

People drive to work rather than walk or bike, take elevators instead of stairs, use dryers rather than hang clothes outside, and cut the lawn with riding mowers rather than with push mowers.

All these modern conveniences reduce the amount of energy expended daily.

Americans are also less active during their leisure time because busy schedules and long days at work and commuting leave little time for active recreation.

Instead, at the end of the day, people tend to sit in front of television sets, video games, tablets, and computers.

Inactivity is also contributing to excess body weight among children. In the 1960s, schools provided daily physical education classes, and children spent their after-school hours playing outdoors; today, they are more likely to spend their afternoons indoors watching television, texting with friends, and playing video games.

As a result, they burn fewer calories, snack more, and consequently gain weight. In the United States, about 17% of children and adolescents ages 2 through 19 are obese,

How energy is released.

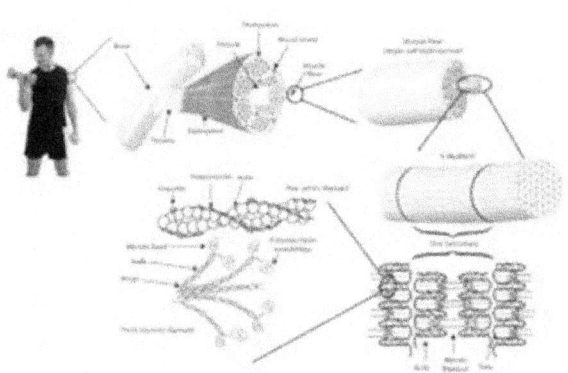

When you need energy, cells release chemical energy from glucose. You need food energy to run, walk and even sleep. Your cells use energy from food to carry out all of their activities.

*Chapter Three ...

Energy Balance – Intake & Expenditure!*

****

The energy needed to fuel your body comes from the food you eat and the energy stored in your body. You use this energy to stay alive, process your food, move, and grow.

Energy balance: Energy In & Energy Out

What you weigh is determined by the balance between how much energy you take in and how much energy you expend.

The Basics of Weight Gain & Weight Loss

If you consume *more* Energy than you *expend*, the *excess* Energy is *stored* for later use – Potential Energy. A small amount of the energy is stored as Glycogen in Liver and Muscle, but most is stored as Triglycerides in **Adipocytes**, which make up adipose tissue. Adipocytes contain large Fat Droplets.

The Cells increase in size as they accumulate more Fat, and they shrink as Fat is removed. If intake *exceeds* needs over the long term, Adipocytes *enlarge*, and the amount of body Fat *increases*, causing weight gain. The larger the number of Adipocytes, the greater the body's ability to *store* Fat.

Most Adipocytes are formed during infancy and adolescence, ***but excessive weight gain can cause the formation of new adipocytes at any time of life***.

Adipocyte - A Cell that stores Fat.

Energy balance: Storing and Retrieving Energy

When calories are consumed in excess of needs, they are stored, mostly as fat. If the excess calories are consumed as fat, they are easily stored as body fat. If the excess calories are consumed as carbohydrate, they are stored as glycogen or converted into fat. If excess calories are consumed as protein, they are converted into body fat.

When calorie intake is less than needs, energy can be retrieved from stores. Glycogen and body proteins can be broken down to supply glucose, and triglycerides in adipose tissue can be broken down to supply fatty acids.

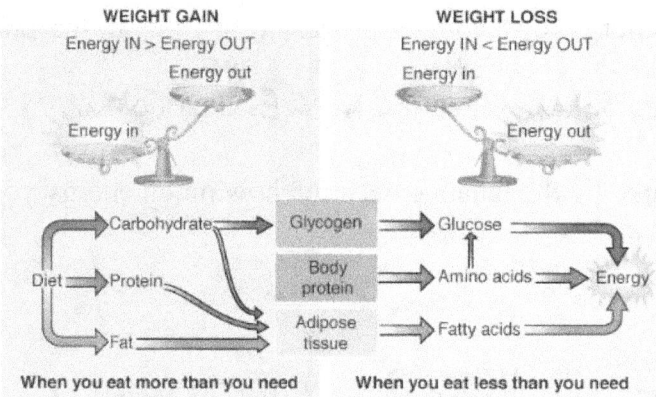

Energy Intake

The amount of energy you consume depends on what and how much you eat and drink. The carbohydrate, fat, protein, and alcohol consumed in food and drink all contribute energy: 4, 9, 4, and 7 Calories/gram, respectively.

Vitamins, Minerals, and Water, though Essential Nutrients, <u>do not</u> provide Energy. Which is why eating for Vitamins and Minerals doesn't increase Energy Levels and after eating you remain tired or become immediately sleepy.

You can determine your calorie intake by using food labels or looking up values in a food composition table or database.

The number of calories in a food depends on the Amount of Carbohydrates, Fats, and Proteins it contains.

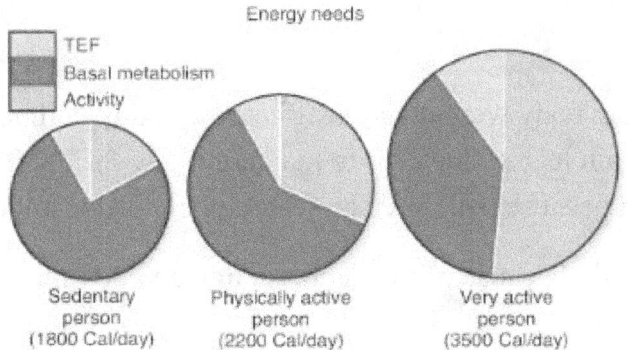

The Amount of energy used to process the food we eat varies with the size and composition of the meal. A bigger meal requires more energy to process so has a higher TEF. A high-fat meal yields a lower TEF than one of similar size that is high in carbohydrate or protein because dietary fat is used and stored more efficiently.

The total amount of energy used by the body each day is referenced as ***Total Energy Expenditure.*** It includes the Energy needed to maintain basic body functions as well as that needed to fuel physical activity and process food. In individuals who are growing or pregnant, Total Energy Expenditure also includes the energy used to deposit new tissues. In women who are lactating, it includes the energy used to produce milk.

A small amount of Energy is also used to maintain our body temperature in a cold environment.

For most people, about 60 to 75% of their Total Energy Expenditure is used for **Basal Metabolism**. This Basal Metabolism includes all our essential metabolic reactions and life-sustaining functions needed to keep us alive, such as breathing, circulating blood, regulating body temperature, synthesizing tissues, removing waste products, and sending nerve signals. The rate at which energy is used for these basic functions is the **Basal Metabolic Rate (BMR)**. This Energy that is expended for Basal Metabolism does *not* include the energy needed for performing physical activities or for the digestion of food and absorption of Nutrients.

Basal Metabolism- The Energy expended to maintain us being awake and a resting body that is not digesting food.

Basal Metabolic Rate (BMR)- The rate of Energy expenditure under Resting conditions. It is measured after 12 hours *without* food or exercise.

BMR increases with increasing body weight and is affected by body composition because it takes more energy to maintain lean tissue than to maintain body fat. BMR is generally higher in men than in women because men have a greater amount of lean body mass.

BMR decreases with age, partly because of the decrease in lean body mass that occurs as we get older.

BMR is also lower when the calorie intake is consistently below the body's needs. This drop in BMR reduces the amount of Energy needed to maintain the body weight. It is a beneficial adaptation in someone who is starving, but in someone who is trying to lose weight, it is frustrating because it makes weight loss more difficult.

Physical activity is the second major component of our Total Energy Expenditure. In most people, physical activity accounts for a smaller proportion of Total Energy Expenditure, more so than Basal Metabolism does—about 15 to 30% of energy requirements.

The Energy we expend in physical activity includes both planned exercise and daily activities such as walking to work, typing, performing yard work, work-related activities, and even fidgeting. This Non-Exercise Activity Thermogenesis (NEAT) includes the energy expended for everything that is not sleeping, eating, or sports-like exercise. In most people it accounts for the majority of the energy expended for activity and varies enormously, depending on an individual's occupation and daily movements.

The amount of Energy used for activity depends on the size of the person, how strenuous the activity is, and the length of time it is performed. Because it takes more energy to move a heavier object, the amount of energy expended for many activities increases as body weight increases. More strenuous activities, such as jogging, use more energy than do less strenuous activities, such as walking, but if you walk for an hour, you will probably burn as many calories as you would by jogging for 30 minutes.

We also use Energy to digest food and to Absorb, Metabolize, and Store the Nutrients from this food. The Energy used for these processes is called either the **Thermic Effect of Food (TEF)** or Diet-induced Thermogenesis.

This energy expenditure causes our Body Temperature to rise slightly for several hours after we have eaten. The energy required for TEF is estimated to be about 10% of energy intake but can vary, depending on the amounts and types of nutrients consumed.

This underscores the importance of our choices and preparation of the foods we choose to consume. This should also lay stress on growing our own food to ensure that we can extract the Highest Quantity and Best Quality of Life Energy possible.

Thermic Effect of Food (TEF) or **Diet-Induced Thermogenesis** = The Energy required for the Digestion of food and Absorption, Metabolism, and Storage of Nutrients.

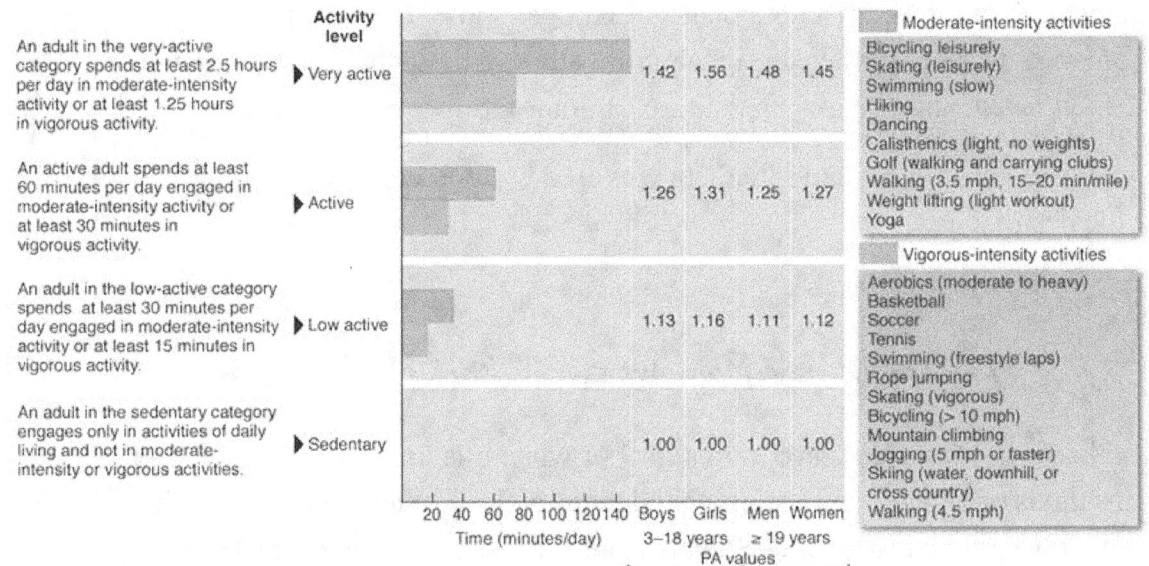

Each physical activity level is assigned a numerical physical activity (PA) value that can then be used in the EER calculation.

Regulation of Food Intake and Body Weight

What we eat and how much we exercise vary from day to day, but body weight tends to stay relatively constant for long periods. Our bodies can compensate for variations in diet and exercise by adjusting energy intake and expenditure to keep weight at a particular level, or *Set Point*.

This Set Point, which is believed to be determined in part by our Genes, explains why your weight can remain fairly constant despite the added activity of a weekend hiking trip, or why most people gain back the weight they lose when they follow a weight-loss diet.

In order for our bodies to Regulate Weight and Fatness at a constant level, the body must be able to respond both to short-term changes in food intake and to long-term changes in the amount of stored body Fat.

Signals related to food intake affect our states of Hunger and **Satiety** over a short period—from meal to meal—whereas signals from adipose tissue trigger the Brain to adjust both food intake and energy expenditure for long-term weight regulation.

Satiety- The feeling of fullness and satisfaction caused by food consumption that eliminates the desire to eat.

Regulating How Much We Eat At Each Meal

How do you know how much to eat for breakfast or when it is time to eat lunch? The physical sensations of Hunger and Satiety that determine how much you eat at each meal are triggered by Neural and Hormonal Signals from the Gastrointestinal Tract, levels of Nutrients and Hormones circulating in the Blood, and messages from the Brain.

Some signals are sent *before* you eat to tell you that you are hungry, some are sent while food is in the Gastrointestinal Tract, and some occur when nutrients are circulating in the Bloodstream.

Regulating How Much We Weigh Over The Long Term

Sometimes we don't pay attention to how full we are after a meal, and we make room for dessert anyway. If this happens often enough, it can cause an increase in body weight and fatness.

To return fatness to a set level, the body must be able to monitor how much fat is present. Some of this information comes from hormones.

Leptin is a good example of a body Hormone that can regulate our level of body fatness in the long term. Leptin is produced by the Adipocytes and the amount produced is directly proportional to the Size of the Adipocytes, and the effect of Leptin on Energy Intake and Expenditure depends on the Amount released.

Unfortunately, Leptin regulation, like other regulatory mechanisms, is much better at preventing weight loss than at preventing weight gain. Obese individuals generally have high levels of leptin, but these levels are not effective at reducing calorie intake and increasing energy expenditure.

Leptin and Body Fat

The average person looking at the photo below would probably see a normal mouse and a very fat mouse. A scientist sees a clue to how body weight is regulated.

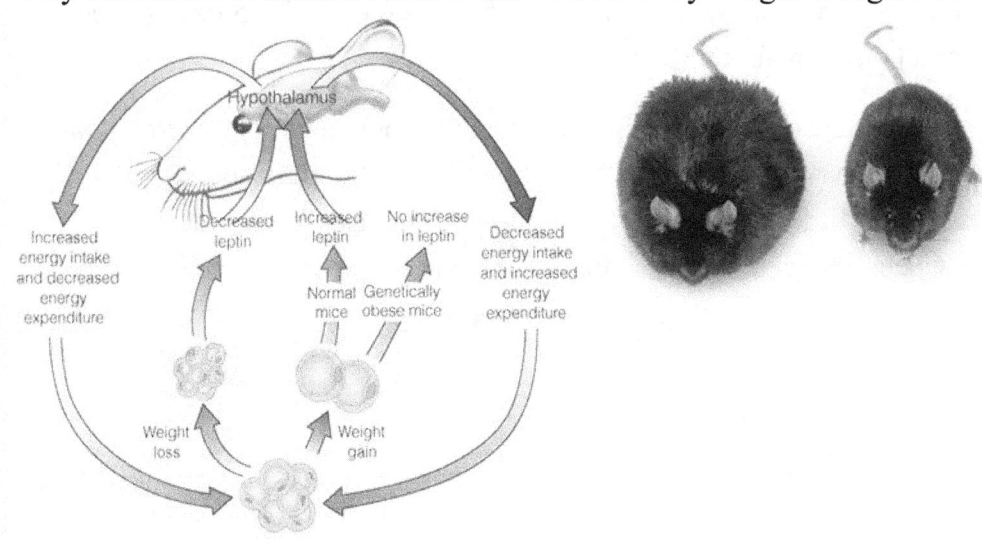

The Hormone Leptin acts in a part of the Brain called the Hypothalamus to help maintain body fat at a normal level.

As expressed in the diagram, the effect of Leptin depends on how much of it is present.

If the mouse *loses* weight, this Fat is lost from the Adipocytes, and *less* Leptin is released as a result, causing an increase in food intake and a decrease in energy expenditure.

If the mouse *gains* weight, then the Adipocytes accumulate Fat, and *more* Leptin is released, resulting in a triggering of events that decrease food intake and increase energy expenditure.

The mouse on the left inherited a defective Leptin Gene, so it produces no Leptin. Even when the Adipocytes enlarge, Leptin levels do not increase. This lack of leptin continues to signal the mouse to eat *more* and expend *less* energy.

The mouse on the right also inherited a defective Leptin Gene, but treatment with Leptin injections returned its weight to normal.

Increasing physical activity

Exercise increases Energy Expenditure and therefore makes weight loss easier. If food intake stays the same, adding enough exercise to expend 200 Calories 5 days a week will result in the loss of a pound in about 3½ weeks.

Exercise also promotes muscle development, and because muscle is metabolically active tissue, increased muscle mass increases Energy Expenditure. In addition, physical activity improves overall fitness and relieves boredom and stress. Weight loss is maintained better when physical activity is included.

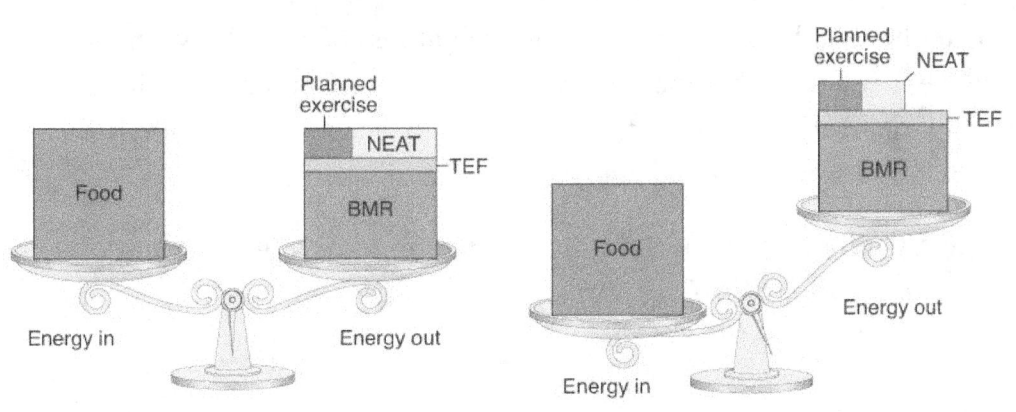

Person 1: Energy balance   Person 2: Weight gain

Modifying Behavior

To successfully lose weight and keep it off, the food consumption and exercise patterns that led to weight gain need to be identified and replaced with new ones that promote and maintain weight loss.

Successful behavior modification includes regular self-monitoring of food intake, physical activity, and weight.

Behavior modification has been shown to effectively help you to establish patterns of food intake and exercise that you can maintain throughout your life without gaining weight.

Diets and Fad Diets

Want to lose 10 lb in just 5 days?   What dieter wouldn't?

People who are desperate to lose weight are prey to all sorts of diets that promise quick fixes. They willingly eat a single food for days at a time, select foods on the basis of special fat-burning qualities, and consume odd combinations at specific times of the day.

Most diets, no matter how outlandish, will promote weight loss because they simple reduce Energy intake. Even diets that focus on modifying Fat or Carbohydrate intake or promise to allow unlimited amounts of certain foods usually accomplish weight loss because the Energy intake is reduced.

The true test of the effectiveness of a weight-loss plan is whether it promotes weight loss that can be maintained over the long term.

Distinguishing between healthy diets and fad diets	
A healthy diet ...	A fad diet ...
Promotes a healthy dietary pattern that meets nutrient needs, includes a variety of foods, suits food preferences, and can be maintained throughout life.	Limits food selections to a few food groups or promotes rituals such as eating only specific food combinations. As a result, it may be limited in certain nutrients and in variety.
Promotes a reasonable weight loss of 0.5 to 2 lb/week and does not restrict energy to under 1200 Cal/day.	Promotes rapid weight loss of much more than 2 lb/week.
Promotes or includes physical activity.	Advertises weight loss without the need to exercise.
Is flexible enough to be followed when eating out and includes foods that are easily obtained.	May require a rigid menu or avoidance of certain foods or may include "magic" foods that promise to burn fat or speed up metabolism.
Does not require costly supplements.	May require the purchase of special foods, weight-loss patches, expensive supplements, creams, or other products.
Promotes a change in behavior. Teaches new eating habits. Provides social support.	Does not recommend changes in activity and eating habits, recommends an eating pattern that is difficult to follow for life, or provides no support other than a book that must be purchased.
Is based on sound scientific principles and may include monitoring by qualified health professionals.	Makes outlandish and unscientific claims, does not support claims that it is clinically tested or scientifically proven, claims that it is new and improved or based on some new scientific discovery, or relies on testimonials from celebrities or connects the diet to trendy places such as Beverly Hills.

People often don't recognize that if you lose weight, you need to eat less to stay at the lower weight.

For example, an inactive 30-year-old, 5′4″ woman who weighs 170 lb needs to consume about 2100 Calories/day to maintain her weight. If she loses 40 lb but does not change her activity level, she will need to consume only about 1880 Calories to maintain her healthier reduced weight. If, once the weight is lost, she resumes her pre-weight-loss dietary pattern, eating 2100 Calories/day, she will regain all the lost weight.

Effective weight-management programs promote healthy weight-loss diets and encourage changes in the lifestyle patterns that led to weight gain.

When selecting a program, look for one that is based on sound nutrition and exercise principles, suits your individual preferences in terms of food choices as well as time and costs, and promotes long-term lifestyle changes.

Quick fixes are tempting, but if the program's approach is not one that can be followed for a lifetime, it is unlikely to promote successful and/or healthy weight management.

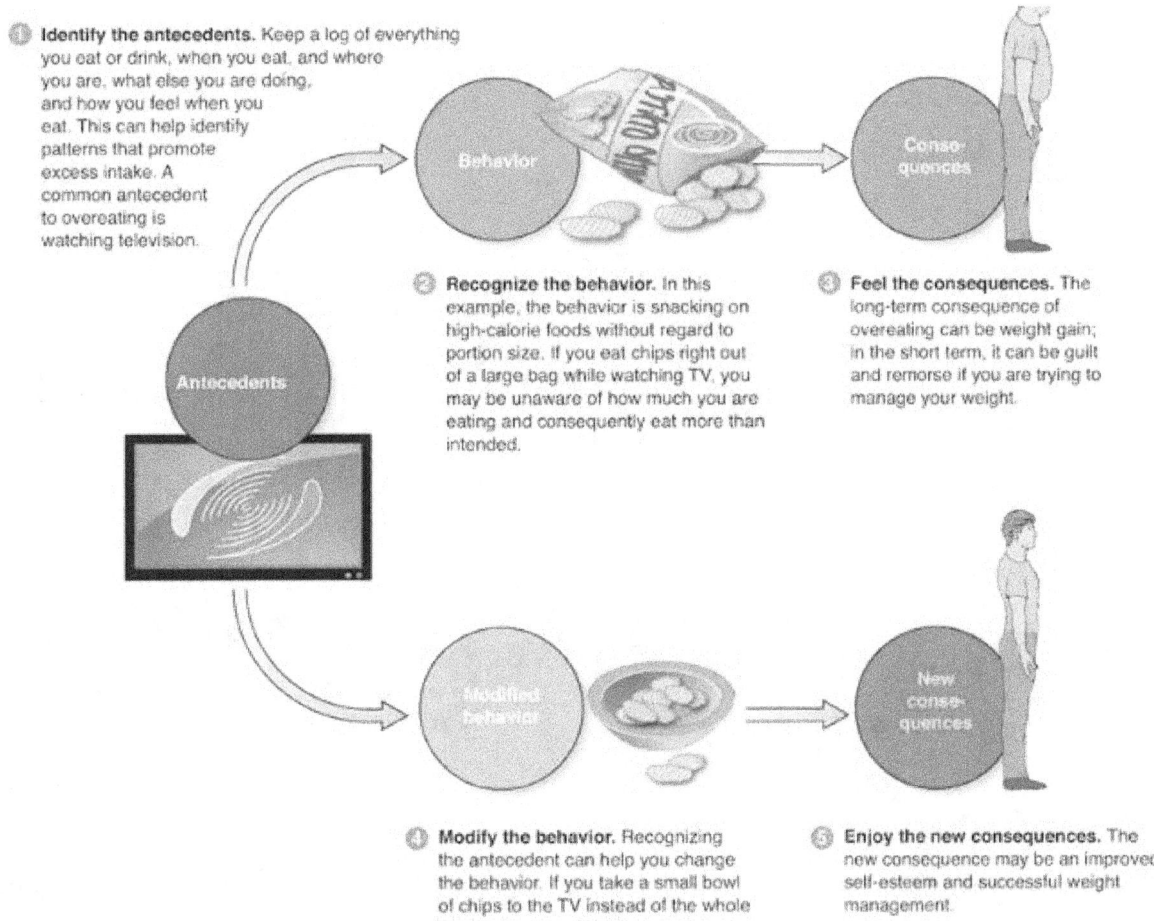

① **Identify the antecedents.** Keep a log of everything you eat or drink, when you eat, and where you are, what else you are doing, and how you feel when you eat. This can help identify patterns that promote excess intake. A common antecedent to overeating is watching television.

② **Recognize the behavior.** In this example, the behavior is snacking on high-calorie foods without regard to portion size. If you eat chips right out of a large bag while watching TV, you may be unaware of how much you are eating and consequently eat more than intended.

③ **Feel the consequences.** The long-term consequence of overeating can be weight gain; in the short term, it can be guilt and remorse if you are trying to manage your weight.

④ **Modify the behavior.** Recognizing the antecedent can help you change the behavior. If you take a small bowl of chips to the TV instead of the whole bag you are less likely to overeat.

⑤ **Enjoy the new consequences.** The new consequence may be an improved self-esteem and successful weight management.

*Chapter Four ...

The Science of Energy/Life Elements*

****

Nutrition builds on two areas of Science. The life sciences of Biochemistry and Physiology details how Nutrition is the catalyst to our physical health and body function. The behavioral sciences help us understand how Nutrition is interwoven with our Psychosocial needs. ***Both of these aspects are at work in our lives***.

Human Organisms are highly complex groupings of Chemical Compounds constantly at work in an array of reactions that sustain life. Nutrients participate in as well as help in the control these Chemical Reactions.

Various Physiologic Systems integrate the activities of millions of functioning cells, uniting them into a functioning whole. This highly sensitive internal control is called **Homeostasis - Homeostatic Control of Energy Balance**.

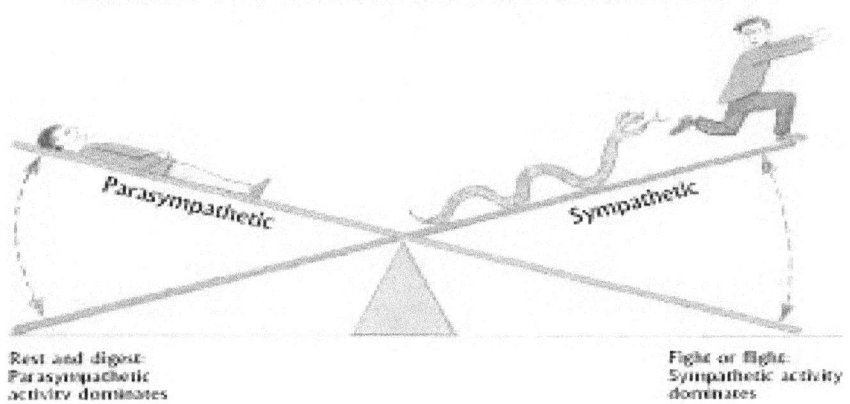

Homeostasis is a dynamic balance between the autonomic branches.

Rest and digest: Parasympathetic activity dominates

Fight or flight: Sympathetic activity dominates

We also have social and emotional qualities rooted in our earliest awareness. Eating patterns and attitudes toward food develop over a lifetime based on the influences of our primary family and friends, ethnic or cultural group, community, nation, and world.

How we perceive food, what we choose to eat, why we eat what we do, and the ways in which we eat are all integral to Human Nutrition.

Our Bodies require many **Nutrients** or Life Elements for the maintenance, growth, and repair of our tissues.

These Nutrients can be divided into six classes: Carbohydrate, Fat, Protein, Vitamins, Minerals, and Water.

The Food and Nutrition Board of the Institute of Medicine has established **Dietary Reference Intakes (DRIs)** to help people achieve a healthy intake of Nutrients.

RECOMMENDED DIETARY INTAKES (RDIS) USED TO ESTABLISH DAILY VALUES

Recommended Dietary Intakes (RDIs)* Used to Establish Daily Values

Source: USDA Food Labeling Guide. Available online at http://www.cfsan.fda.gov/'dms/2lg-xf.htm

Vitamins and Minerals	Units of Measurement	Adults and Children 4 or more Years of Age	Infants	Children Under 4 Years of Age	Pregnant or Lactating Women
Vitamin A	International Units†	5000 (1000 µg)	1500	2500	8000
Vitamin D	International Units†	400 (10 µg)	400	400	400
Vitamin E	International Units†	30 (10 µg)	5	10	30
Vitamin C	Milligrams	60	35	40	60
Folic acid	Micrograms	400	0.1	0.2	0.8
Thiamin	Milligrams	1.5	0.5	0.7	1.7
Riboflavin	Milligrams	1.7	0.6	0.8	2.0
Niacin	Milligrams	20	8	9	20
Vitamin B$_6$	Milligrams	2.0	0.4	0.7	2.5
Vitamin B$_{12}$	Micrograms	6.0	2	3	8
Biotin	Micrograms	300	0.05	0.15	0.30
Pantothenic acid	Milligrams	10	3	5	10
Calcium	Milligrams	1000	0.6	0.8	1.3
Phosphorous	Milligrams	1000	0.5	0.8	1.3
Iodine	Micrograms	150	45	70	150
Iron	Milligrams	18	15	10	18
Magnesium	Milligrams	400	70	200	450
Copper	Milligrams	2.0	0.6	1.0	2.0
Zinc	Milligrams	15	5	8	15
Vitamin K	Micrograms	80	‡	‡	‡
Chromium	Micrograms	120	—	—	—
Selenium	Micrograms	70	—	—	—
Molybdenum	Micrograms	75	—	—	—
Manganese	Milligrams	2	—	—	—
Chloride	Milligrams	3400	—	—	—

*Based on National Academy of Sciences' 1968 Recommended Dietary Allowances.

†The RDIs for fat-soluble vitamins are expressed in International Units (IU). Values that are approximately equivalent in micrograms are given in parentheses.

‡No values yet established for vitamin K, chromium, selenium, molybdenum, manganese, or chloride for this population.

The DRIs consist of recommended intakes for nutrients based on age and sex, including the **Recommended Dietary Allowances** **(RDAs),** or the amounts found to be adequate for approximately 97% of the population; **Adequate Intakes** **(AIs),** or the amounts considered adequate although insufficient data exist to establish the appropriate RDA; and **Tolerable Upper intake Levels** **(UL),** or the highest intakes believed to pose no health risk.

Additionally, **Acceptable Macronutrient Distribution Ranges (AMDRs)** have been established for Carbohydrate, Fat and protein. The Institute of Medicine reports can be accessed at the National Academies Press website (www.nap.edu).

Our body runs on the Energy from the Carbohydrates, Fats, and Protein in our food, and it can also use Energy from our Body stores. These fuels are needed whether you are writing a term paper, riding your bike to class, or running a marathon. Before they can be used to fuel activity, their Energy must be transferred to the High-Energy compound ATP, the immediate source of Energy for body functions.

ATP can be generated both in the absence of Oxygen, by **Anaerobic Metabolism**, and in the presence of Oxygen, by **Aerobic Metabolism**. The type of metabolism that predominates during an activity determines how much Carbohydrate, Fat, and Protein are used to fuel the activity.

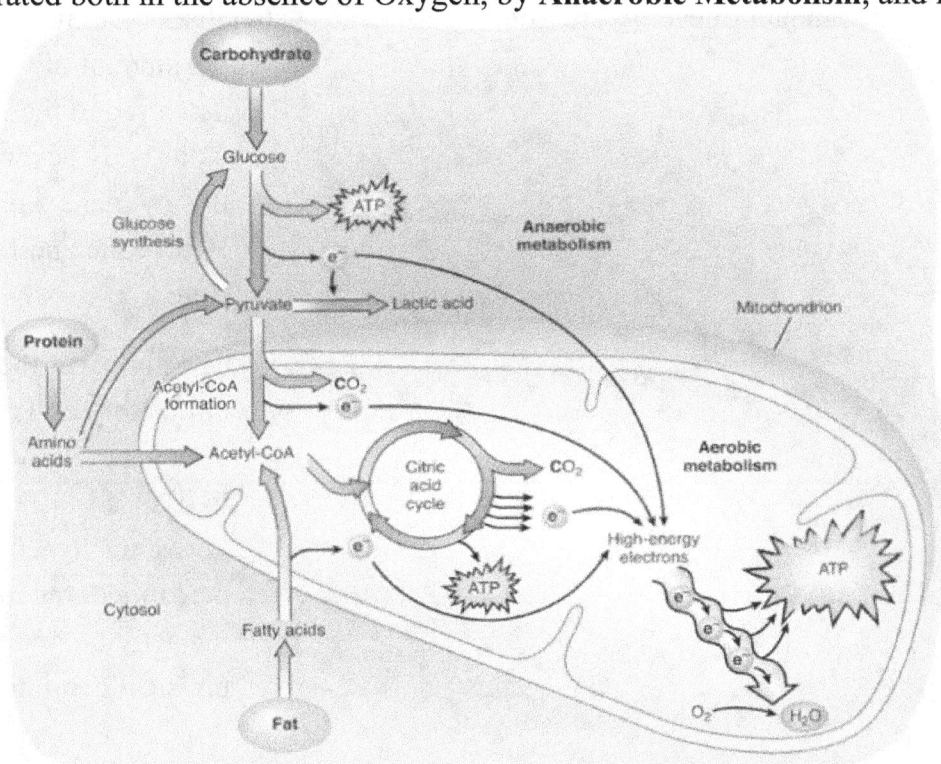

Page / 63

ATP is produced in the Cytosol by Anaerobic metabolism when no oxygen is available.

Anaerobic Metabolism produces ATP very rapidly but uses only glucose as a fuel. The **Lactic Acid** that is produced can be used as a fuel for aerobic metabolism.

Aerobic Metabolism requires Oxygen, takes place in our Mitochondria, and can use Carbohydrates, Fats, or Protein to generate ATP.

Aerobic Metabolism produces the majority of ATP; Aerobic Metabolism is slower but more efficient at generating ATP than with Anaerobic Metabolism.

The availability of Oxygen is the determining factor as to whether ATP is produced predominantly by Anaerobic versus Aerobic metabolism. Oxygen is taken in by our Respiratory system and delivered to our Muscles by our Blood.

When you are at rest, your Muscles do not need much Energy, and your Heart and Lungs are able to deliver enough Oxygen to meet your Energy needs using Aerobic Metabolism. When you exercise, your Muscles need *more* Energy.

To increase the amount of energy provided by Aerobic Metabolism, you must increase the amount of Oxygen delivered to the Muscles. Your body accomplishes this by increasing both Heart Rate and Breathing Rate.

CO_2 O_2
Lungs

⑤ Carbon dioxide is exhaled through the lungs.

CO_2 O_2

① Inhaled oxygen is transferred from the lungs to the blood.

Heart

② The cardiovascular system circulates the oxygen-rich blood throughout the body.

Blood vessels

Muscles ③ Oxygen is taken up by the muscles and other tissues and used to generate ATP, producing carbon dioxide as a waste product.

④ Carbon dioxide is carried away from the muscle by the blood.

The ability of the circulatory and respiratory systems to deliver oxygen to tissues is affected by how long an activity is performed, the intensity of the activity, and the physical conditioning of the exerciser.

Getting Oxygen to Muscle Cells

When you exercise, your Muscles need *more* Oxygen. Your body responds to this need by breathing faster and deeper in order to take in more oxygen through the lungs and by increasing heart rate in order to deliver the additional oxygen to your muscles.

Exercise Duration and Fuel Use

When you take the first steps of your morning jog, your muscles increase their activity, but your heart and lungs have not had time to step up their delivery of Oxygen to them.

To get the Energy they need, the Muscles rely on the small amount of ATP that is stored in Resting Muscle. This is enough to sustain activity for a few seconds. As this stored ATP is used up, Enzymes break-down another High-Energy compound, **Creatine Phosphate**, to convert ADP (Adenosine Di-Phosphate) to ATP, allowing your activity to continue.

But, like the amount of ATP, the amount of Creatine Phosphate stored in the muscle at any time is *small* and soon runs out.

Creatine Phosphate- A compound stored in the Muscle that can be broken down quickly to make ATP.

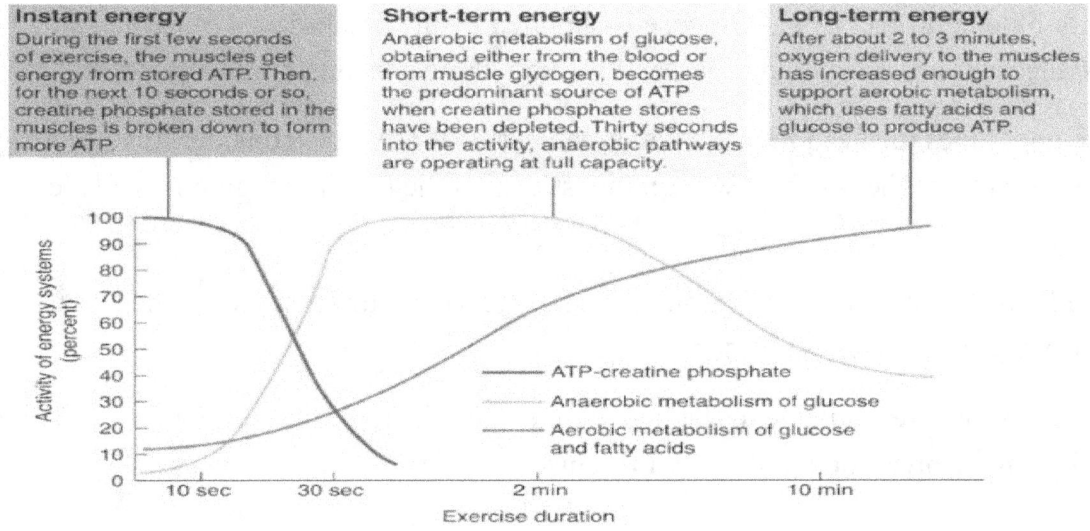

Instant energy During the first few seconds of exercise, the muscles get energy from stored ATP. Then, for the next 10 seconds or so, creatine phosphate stored in the muscles is broken down to form more ATP.

Short-term energy Anaerobic metabolism of glucose, obtained either from the blood or from muscle glycogen, becomes the predominant source of ATP when creatine phosphate stores have been depleted. Thirty seconds into the activity, anaerobic pathways are operating at full capacity.

Long-term energy After about 2 to 3 minutes, oxygen delivery to the muscles has increased enough to support aerobic metabolism, which uses fatty acids and glucose to produce ATP.

ATP-creatine phosphate
Anaerobic metabolism of glucose
Aerobic metabolism of glucose and fatty acids

Activity of energy systems (percent)

Exercise duration

Changes in the source of ATP over time

The source of the ATP that fuels muscle contraction changes over the first few minutes of exercise. If the intensity of activity remains moderate, Aerobic Metabolism will predominate after about 5 minutes.

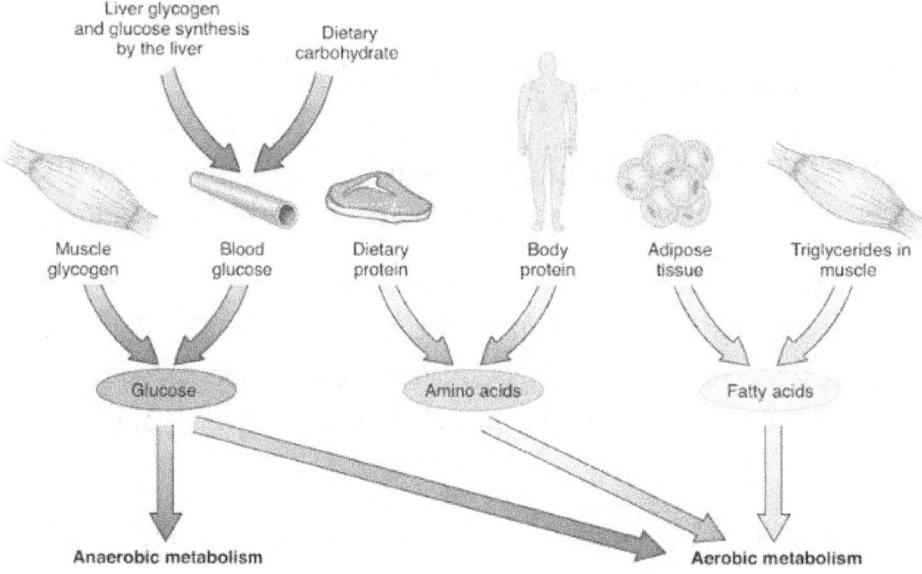

Fuels for Aerobic and Anaerobic Metabolism

The Glucose that is used to Fuel Muscle Contraction comes from muscle glycogen breakdown or blood glucose. Blood Glucose is supplied by the break-down of Liver Glycogen, Glucose synthesis by the Liver, and Carbohydrate consumed in the diet.

This science underlines the need to make better choices of WHAT we consider food, as well as HOW to prepare them so that we can digest/extract the maximum amount of Life Energy.

Some of the Fatty Acids used as fuel come from Triglycerides stored in the Muscle, but most come from those in Adipose Tissue.

The Amino Acids that are available to the body come from the digestion of dietary Proteins and from the break-down of Body Proteins.

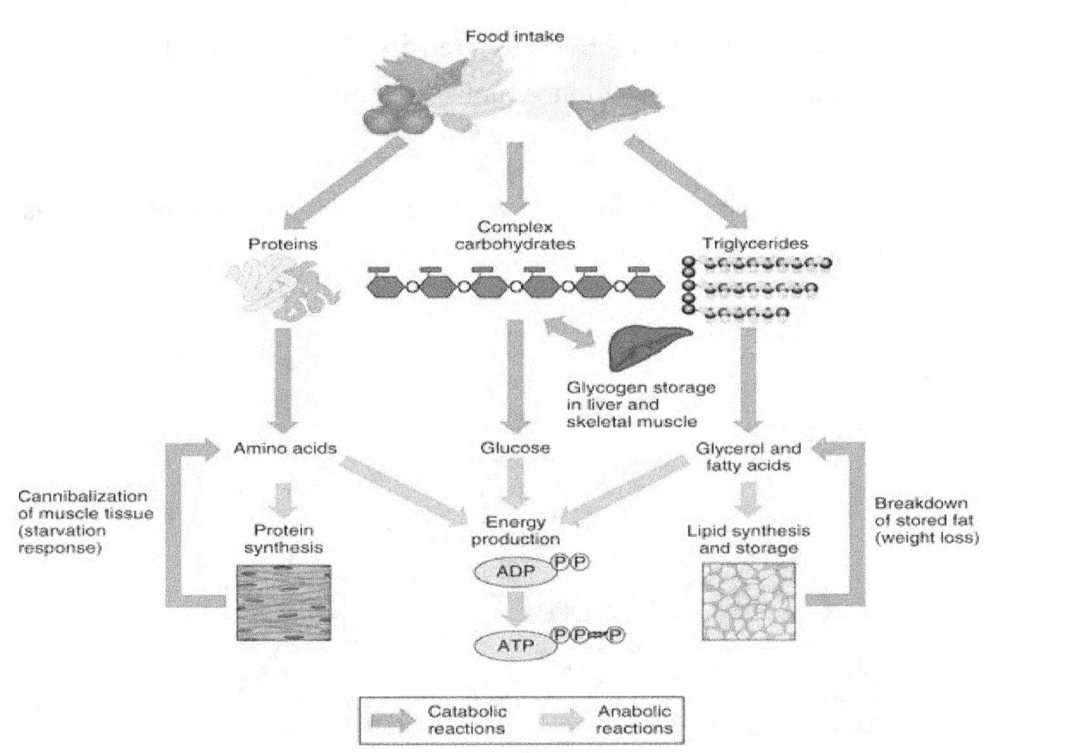

Long-term Energy: Aerobic metabolism

After you have been exercising for 2 to 3 minutes, your breathing and heart rate have increased to supply more Oxygen to your Muscles. This allows Aerobic Metabolism to predominate.

Aerobic metabolism produces ATP at a slower rate than does Anaerobic Metabolism, but it is much more efficient, producing about 18 times more ATP for each Molecule of Glucose.

As a result, Glucose is used more slowly than in Anaerobic Metabolism. In addition, Aerobic Metabolism can use Fatty Acids, and Amino Acids from Protein, which can be used to generate ATP.

In a typical adult, about 90% of Stored Energy is found in the Adipose Tissue; this provides an ample supply of Fatty Acids that can later be used to manifest Energy.

When you continue to exercise at a low to moderate intensity, Aerobic Metabolism predominates, and fatty acids become the primary fuel source for your exercising muscles.

When you pick up the pace, the relative amount of ATP generated by Anaerobic versus Aerobic Metabolism and the fuels you burn will change.

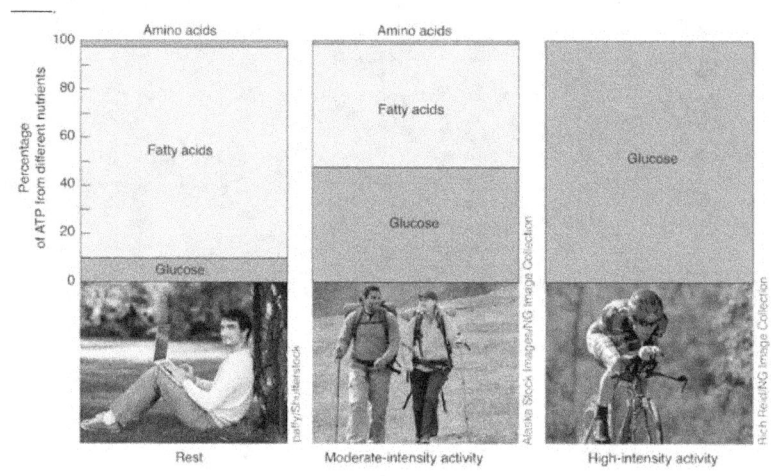

Protein as an Energy Source

Although Protein is not considered as a major Energy source for our bodies, even at rest, small amounts of Amino Acids are used for Energy. The amount increases if your diet does **_not_** provide enough Total Energy to meet needs, if you consume *more* Protein than you need, or if you are involved in endurance exercise.

Understanding our Human Energy needs allows us to eat according to our Anatomical structure and function, in-turn giving us the best results to successfully manifest the Highest Quality and Expression of Humanity = The Direct Express Image & Likeness of The CREATOR!

When the Nitrogen-containing amino group is removed from an amino acid, the remaining carbon compound can be broken down to produce ATP by Aerobic Metabolism or, in some cases, used to make Glucose.

Exercise that continues for many hours increases the use of amino acids both as an energy source and as a raw material for Glucose synthesis.

*Strength training does **not** increase the use of Protein for energy, but it does increase the demand for Amino Acids for the building and repair of Muscle tissue.*

Effect of Exercise Intensity on Energy Use

Exercise intensity determines the contributions of Carbohydrates, Fats, and Protein needed as fuels for ATP production.

At rest and during low- to moderate-intensity exercise, Aerobic Metabolism predominates, so Fatty Acids become an important fuel source.

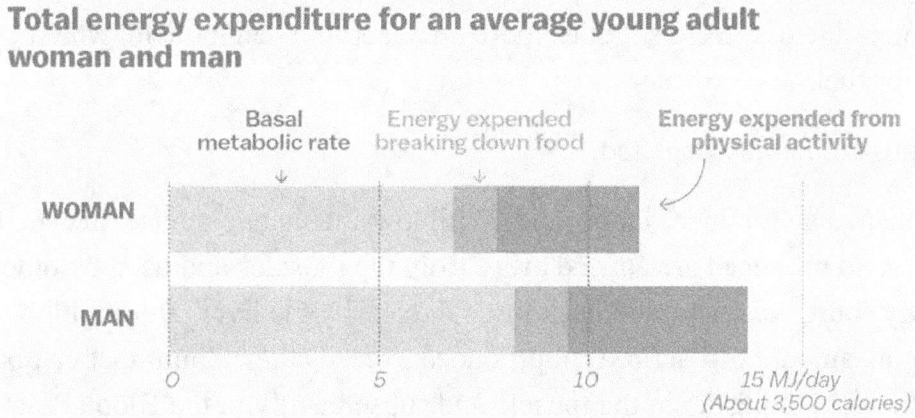

Total energy expenditure for an average young adult woman and man

As exercise intensity increases, the proportion of energy supplied by anaerobic metabolism increases, so glucose becomes the predominant fuel.

Keep in mind, however, that during exercise, the total amount of Energy expended is greater than the amount expended at rest, which make proper food choices and preparation even more imp0rtant to maintain adequate Energy Balance and successfully achieve Homeostasis.

Lower-intensity exercise relies predominantly on Aerobic Metabolism, which is more efficient than Anaerobic Metabolism as well as utilizing both Glucose and Fatty Acids to produce ATP.

Our body's fat reserves are almost unlimited, so if Fat is the fuel, exercise can theoretically continue for a very long time.

For example, it is estimated that a 130-pound woman has enough Energy stored as body Fat to run 1000 miles.

However, even Aerobic activity uses some Glucose, which means that if exercise continues long enough, Glycogen stores are eventually depleted, causing Fatigue.

Fatigue has many causes, including Glycogen depletion, increased Muscle Acidity, and other changes in the Muscle Cells and the concentrations of Molecules involved in Muscle Metabolism.

Fatigue occurs much more quickly with high-intensity exercise than with lower-intensity exercise because more intense exercise relies more on anaerobic metabolism, which can use only Glucose for fuel.

Glycogen stores thus are rapidly depleted.

Anaerobic metabolism also produces lactic acid. With low-intensity exercise, the small amounts of Lactic Acid produced are carried away from the muscles and used by other tissues as an Energy source or converted back into Glucose by the liver. During high-intensity exercise, the amount of Lactic Acid produced exceeds the amount that can be used, and the Lactic Acid builds up in the muscle and subsequently in the Blood. Lactic Acid buildup accompanies exercise-associated Muscle fatigue, but it is still not known to what extent Lactic Acid causes Fatigue.

ELEMENTS OF LIFE

- 96% of living organisms are made of:
  1. **Carbon** (C)
  2. **Oxygen** (O)
  3. **Hydrogen** (H)
  4. **Nitrogen** (N)

And also …

  5. **Sulfur** (S)
  6. **Phosphate** (P)

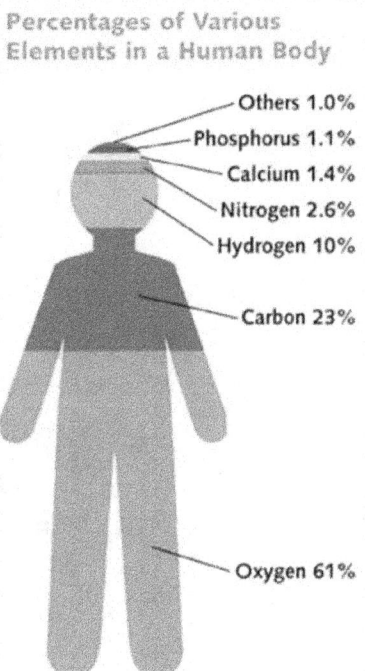

Percentages of Various Elements in a Human Body

Others 1.0%
Phosphorus 1.1%
Calcium 1.4%
Nitrogen 2.6%
Hydrogen 10%
Carbon 23%
Oxygen 61%

*Chapter Five ....

Body Composition!*

*****

Finding a Healthy Weight

Nothing is more personal than your own body. And nothing has a greater influence over how long that body functions properly than its composition.

Body composition is the ratio of Muscle Mass to Fat Mass.

Muscle mass is composed of Muscle, Bone, Organs, and other Tissues of the body.

Fat mass is the total amount of Essential and Storage Fat in the body.

BMI	Classification
Less than 18.5	Underweight
18.5—24.9	Normal
25—29.9	Overweight
30—34.9	Mildly Obese
35.0—39.9	Moderately Obese
40 or greater	Severely Obese

Essential Body Fat

Page | 73

Your **Essential Body Fat** resides in your Nerve Cells, Muscles, and Bone Marrow, as well as in your Lungs, Heart, Liver, and Intestines.

It has many important functions:

■ Keeps your physiological activity normal (e.g., nerve conduction)

■ Helps keep your body warm

■ Protects your organs from injury

■ Stores energy needed when your body is active or when you are injured or ill

The desirable amount of essential fat for a healthy person is:

■ Adult women: 8% to 12% of total body weight

■ Adult men: 3% to 5% of total body weight

Women have more essential body Fat in their Hips, Thighs, Breasts, and Uterus.

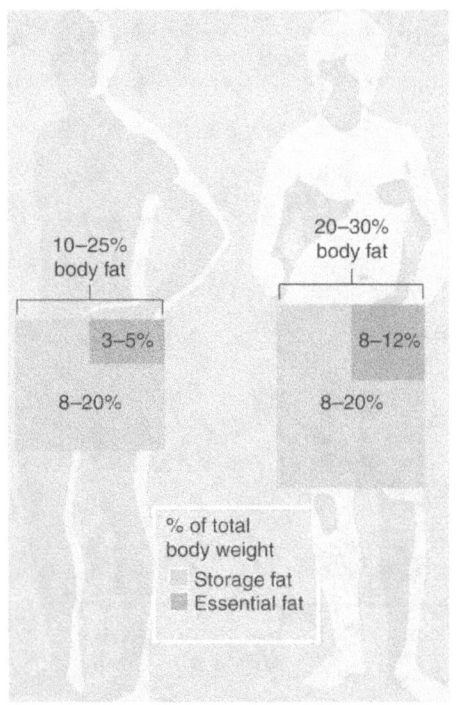

10–25% body fat

20–30% body fat

3–5%

8–12%

8–20%

8–20%

% of total body weight
Storage fat
Essential fat

Storage Fat

A small amount of Fat beyond what is Essential is also desirable in survival or emergency situations. Besides organ protection and body insulation, **Storage Fat** supplies Energy: approximately 3500 calories per pound of Adipose Tissue.

A variety of methods exist for determining whether body composition places a person at risk for disease.

Some methods are simple calculations and are based on the relationship between the person's height and weight. Other methods look specifically at the fat contained in the body.

For many people a normal body weight cannot be defined. In the traditional sense, being overweight and/or excessive body Fat simply represent an Energy imbalance arising from a surplus in Energy Input (Eating) over Energy Output (Total Energy Expenditure).

But it is also not that simple. Our genetic makeup influences our propensity to weight gain and the amount and position of body fat as well as our ability to control and/or lose it.

Estrogen and Testosterone control the differences in body Fat between men and women, but other internal mechanisms also lead to differences in fat accretion. Certain individuals have an exceptionally low RMR and a High Metabolic Efficiency influenced by an inherited obesity Gene, which adds to their risk of unwanted weight.

A genetic link has been identified among certain Native Americans that characterizes their lower energy expenditure and higher BMI and contributes to their elevated risk for Type-2 diabetes. Fidgeting and ongoing body movement, sometimes referred to as ***Non-Exercise Activity Thermogenesis*** (NEAT) increases energy expenditure and helps some people resist weight gain even if overfed.

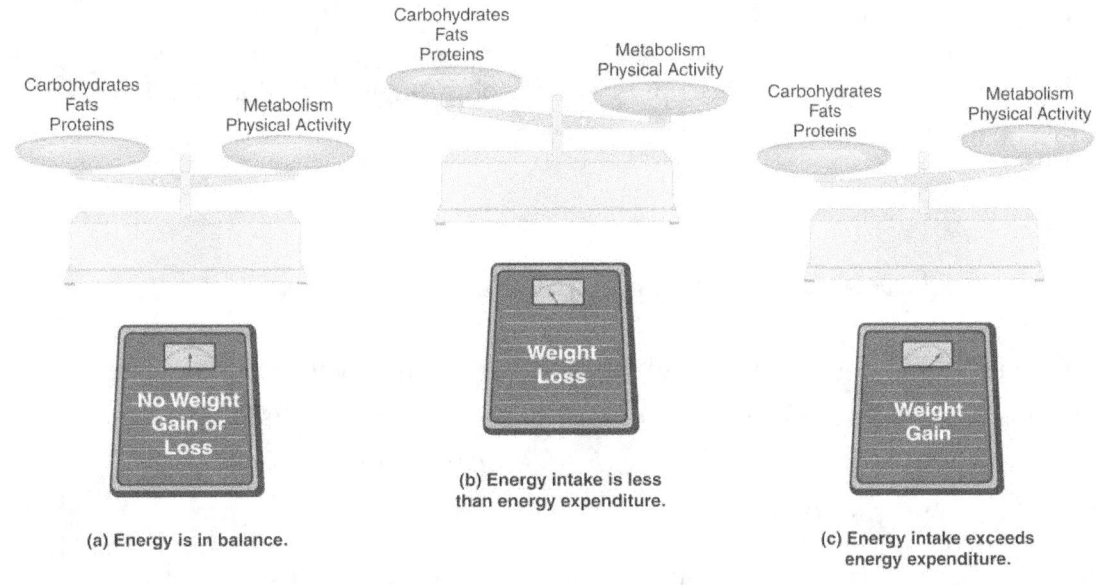

(a) Energy is in balance.

(b) Energy intake is less than energy expenditure.

(c) Energy intake exceeds energy expenditure.

Just as weight gain results from a surplus of kcalories, weight loss should follow a kcalorie deficit. Traditionally it was believed that a shortfall of 3500 kcal would bring about the loss of 1 lb of body weight; however, this can be a false promise, and leading clinicians recommend that it not be used.

Body mechanisms designed to preserve body mass can decrease spontaneous activity or lower the RMR, making weight loss more difficult. When weight loss is successful, RMR and energy requirements decrease as body tissue is lost.

Adding an exercise component assists in weight management if individuals do not increase their energy intake as a result of the activity.

For some individuals the weight loss required to move them into a more appropriate weight range is not possible. Yet, it is critical to interrupt a cycle of continued weight gain.

The American Heart Association points to the misperception created by an emphasis on body weight and mortality.

Although body weight in the overweight or moderately obese range does not always result in earlier death, even small increases in body weight can add to risk of chronic conditions that adversely affect quality of life.

Conversely, small losses in body weight interrupt or slow such changes. So what should be our approach to a healthy weight?

Developing a Healthy Lifestyle

The goals of weight management go well beyond numbers on a scale, even if a change in weight is one of the objectives. ***Successful weight management requires a lifelong commitment to positive lifestyle behaviors that emphasize sustainable and enjoyable eating habits and daily physical activity.***

A healthy food and activity pattern is a more appropriate goal than weight loss at any cost. A meal plan low to moderate in Fat and rich in Fruits, Veggies, Whole Grains, and

Fiber at an Energy level that prevents further weight gain adds to well-being regardless of weight loss.

Regular physical activity such as walking lowers the risk of heart attack, even if individuals remain obese. A stable weight, even if above desirable weight, is favored over regular cycles of weight loss followed by even greater weight gain.

Page / 76

Body Composition: Fatness and Leanness

A person's body composition reflects his or her total lifetime Nutrient and Energy Balance. Individuals have different body shapes and sizes depending on their age, gender, genes, body type, and state of health.

Ectomorphs have a body type that is generally slender and fragile, mesomorphs have prominent muscle and bone development, and endomorphs have a soft, round physique with some accumulation of body fat.

Although each body type has a genetic base, dietary intake and physical activity influence how it is expressed. Some body types are associated with better health, whereas others carry increased risk of chronic disease. We need to be sensitive to different body types when developing strategies to improve body composition and health.

Cell membrane
Cytoplasm
Nucleus
Fat droplet

The number of fat cells increases in normal growth

In obese people, fat cells are larger than in lean people

Fat cells divide when they reach a certain size

With fat loss, the size of the cells, but not the number, decreases

Body Weight & Body Fat
Overweight Vs Overfat

Because height and weight are easily measured, they are commonly used to assess health status.

It is important to know what these measurements do and do not tell us.

Adult Females				
Age	Increased Risk	Healthy	Increased Risk	Greatly Increased Risk
20–39	Less than 21%	21% to 32%	33% to 38%	Over 39%
40–59	Less than 23%	23% to 33%	34% to 39%	Over 40%
60–79	Less than 24%	24% to 35%	36% to 41%	Over 42%

Adult Males				
Age	Increased Risk	Healthy	Increased Risk	Greatly Increased Risk
20–39	Less than 8%	8% to 19%	20% to 24%	Over 25%
40–59	Less than 11%	11% to 21%	22% to 27%	Over 28%
60–79	Less than 13%	13% to 24%	24% to 29%	Over 30%

The terms *over-weight* and *obesity* have different meanings as related to body composition, and these distinctions have implications for health.

A football player in peak physical condition can be markedly "overweight" according to standard height-weight charts. That is, the player weighs more than the average person of similar height, but that player's body tissues are likely to be very different.

A sedentary man above average weight likely has an excess amount of body fat that is adding to his total body weight; an athlete above average weight is likely to have an exceptionally large amount of muscle.

In fact, the overweight athlete may have an even lower proportion of body fat than an individual of average weight.

When overweight is the result of Excessive Body Fat rather than enhanced Muscle or Skeletal Tissue – *over-fat* or *obese* is the appropriate term.

The critical element when evaluating body build and health is body composition.

What we really need to know is how much of a person's body weight is Fat and how much is *Fat-Free Mass* (FFM).

It is more precise to think in terms of *fatness* and *leanness* rather than body weight or overweight.

Body Compartments

Body compartments are defined on the basis of their comparative size and metabolic activity. The relative amounts of specific body tissues sometimes overlap among compartments.

The four-compartment model for evaluating body composition includes Lean Body Mass (LBM), Body Fat, Body Water, and Mineral Mass, as follows:

1. **_LBM_**: This compartment is made up of active cells from muscle and vital organs and largely determines the BMR and related nutrient needs. In sedentary individuals it accounts for almost the entire energy requirement. LBM includes not only Cell Protein but also a large amount of water, because Muscle Cells are about 65% water. This compartment also contains very small amounts of fatty acids found in the membranes of muscle and organ cells. LBM changes in size across the life cycle, with steady growth through childhood and young adulthood and gradual loss in later years. In adults it makes up 30% to 65% of total body weight.

Most weight reduction regimens result in a loss of both body fat and LBM. (LBM contains cell protein, cell water, and a very small amount of fat found in membranes, while FFM includes cell protein, all body water both inside and outside of cells, and bone mineral mass—all body tissues except for fat.)

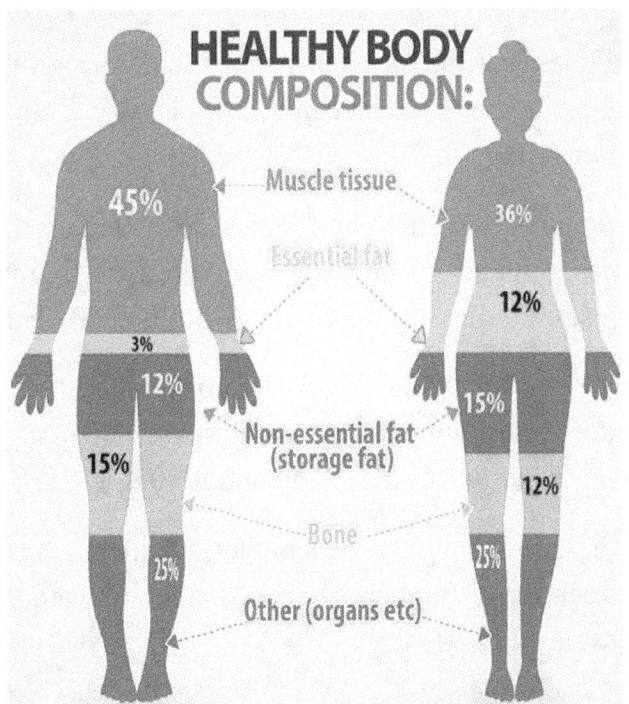

2. **_Body fat_**: Total body fat reflects both the number and size of the Fat Cells (**adipocytes**) that form the Adipose tissue.

Most Adipocytes are White Fat Cells, not the brown fat cells we referred to earlier.

In an adult man of normal weight, fat comprises 13% to 21% of body weight. In a woman of normal weight, the range of body fat content is 23% to 31%.

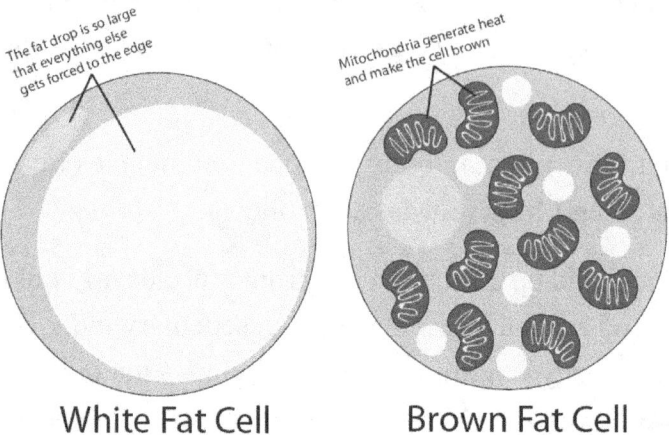

The fat drop is so large that everything else gets forced to the edge

Mitochondria generate heat and make the cell brown

White Fat Cell   Brown Fat Cell

These amounts vary with age, body type, exercise, and fitness, and many people have body fat levels markedly greater than or less than these ranges. About one half of all body fat is located in the subcutaneous fat layers under the skin, where it serves as insulation. In children and young adults, the subcutaneous fat provides a useful measure for estimating total body fat.

Skinfold thickness measured at various locations on the body such as the triceps, subscapular region, or waist can be applied to existing standards to assess relative leanness or fatness.

As individuals grow older, body fat is deposited on the trunk rather than on the extremities; thus waist circumference, waist-to-hip ratio, and waist-to-height ratio become useful tools to evaluate body fatness and health risk.

3. **_Body water_**_:_ Total body water includes both intracellular and extracellular water. Total body water varies with relative leanness or fatness, age, hydration status, and health status. Generally, water makes up about 50% to 65% of body weight.

 Muscle Tissue has *high* water content, whereas Adipose Tissue has *low* water content; therfore men have a higher proportion of body water than women because they have *more* muscle and *less* fat.

Infants have a relatively high proportion of body water, which drops to adult levels by age 2. This makes them especially vulnerable to the dangers of dehydration with continued vomiting or diarrhea.

4. *__Mineral mass__*: Body minerals found largely in the skeleton account for only 4% to 6% of body weight. Major minerals are calcium and phosphorus located in bone and other body cells and in fluids. Sodium is the major mineral in extracellular fluid (ECF), and potassium is the major mineral in intracellular fluid (ICF).

The following factors influence the relative sizes of body compartments:

• *Gender:* Women have more adipose tissue, and men have more lean tissue, particularly muscle tissue.

• *Age:* Young adults have more LBM and less fat than older adults.

• *Physical activity:* Persons who are physically active have less fat and more LBM than individuals who are sedentary.

• *Race:* African Americans have relatively more bone mineral than Caucasians or Hispanics; Caucasian men tend to have more body fat than African-American men of similar height and weight; Mexican-American women tend to have more body fat than African-American women with similar heights and weights.

• *Climate:* Individuals living in very cold climates develop more subcutaneous fat to insulate against heat loss.

Importance of Body Fat

Although excess body fat is detrimental to health, some body fat is necessary for life. In human starvation, victims die from Fat *LOSS* and *NOT* Protein depletion. For mere survival, men require about 3% body Fat and women require about 12%; however, for reproductive capacity women require a body Fat of about 20%.

Theories of Weight Gain

Fat Cell Theory

Fat cell theory says that obesity is related to too many fat cells and enlarged fat cells. People with an above-average number of fat cells may have been born with them or may have developed them at certain times because of overeating. Restricting calories decreases only the size of fat cells, not the number.

Set Point Theory

Set Point theory states that obese individuals are "programmed" to carry a certain amount of weight. This programming originates from a weight regulatory mechanism in the Brain's Hypothalamus. Even if you lose weight, your body strives to get back to its set point. To lose weight, you must change the set point.

Glandular Disorder Theory

Hypothyroidism is seldom the main reason for overweight or obesity. Treatment with a Thyroid Hormone, although medically unnecessary, does not usually cause a significant weight reduction.

Genetics

More than 400 different Genes have been implicated in the development of overweight or obesity, although only a handful appear to be major players. Genes contribute to obesity in many ways, such as by affecting appetite, satiety (the sense of fullness), metabolism, food cravings, body fat distribution, and the tendency to use eating as a way to cope with stress.

The initiation of Menstruation or **Menarche** occurs when the female body attains a certain size or, more precisely, the critical proportion of body Fat.

Body fat gained during pregnancy serves as an important energy reserve for lactation, and the production of breast milk with its high energy cost usually brings about a gradual loss of these fat stores.

Ill-advised dieting during pregnancy in an attempt to avoid normal weight gain interferes with fetal development and can result in a low–birth-weight infant with associated health risks.

	Normal						Overweight					Obese									Extreme Obesity															
BMI	19	20	21	22	23	24	25	26	27	28	29	30	31	32	33	34	35	36	37	38	39	40	41	42	43	44	45	46	47	48	49	50	51	52	53	54
Height (inches)															Body Weight (pounds)																					
58	91	96	100	105	110	115	119	124	129	134	138	143	148	153	158	162	167	172	177	181	186	191	196	201	205	210	215	220	224	229	234	239	244	248	253	258
59	94	99	104	109	114	119	124	128	133	138	143	148	153	158	163	168	173	178	183	188	193	198	203	208	212	217	222	227	232	237	242	247	252	257	262	267
60	97	102	107	112	118	123	128	133	138	143	148	153	158	163	168	174	179	184	189	194	199	204	209	215	220	225	230	235	240	245	250	255	261	266	271	276
61	100	106	111	116	122	127	132	137	143	148	153	158	164	169	174	180	185	190	195	201	206	211	217	222	227	232	238	243	248	254	259	264	269	275	280	285
62	104	109	115	120	126	131	136	142	147	153	158	164	169	175	180	186	191	196	202	207	213	218	224	229	235	240	246	251	256	262	267	273	278	284	289	295
63	107	113	118	124	130	135	141	146	152	158	163	169	175	180	186	191	197	203	208	214	220	225	231	237	242	248	254	259	265	270	278	282	287	293	299	304
64	110	116	122	128	134	140	145	151	157	163	169	174	180	186	192	197	204	209	215	221	227	232	238	244	250	256	262	267	273	279	285	291	296	302	308	314
65	114	120	126	132	138	144	150	156	162	168	174	180	186	192	198	204	210	216	222	228	234	240	246	252	258	264	270	276	282	288	294	300	306	312	318	324
66	118	124	130	136	142	148	155	161	167	173	179	186	192	198	204	210	216	223	229	235	241	247	253	260	266	272	278	284	291	297	303	309	315	322	328	334
67	121	127	134	140	146	153	159	166	172	178	185	191	198	204	211	217	223	230	236	242	249	255	261	268	274	280	287	293	299	306	312	319	325	331	338	344
68	125	131	138	144	151	158	164	171	177	184	190	197	203	210	216	223	230	236	243	249	256	262	269	276	282	289	295	302	308	315	322	328	335	341	348	354
69	128	135	142	149	155	162	169	176	182	189	196	203	209	216	223	230	236	243	250	257	263	270	277	284	291	297	304	311	318	324	331	338	345	351	358	365
70	132	139	146	153	160	167	174	181	188	195	202	209	216	222	229	236	243	250	257	264	271	278	285	292	299	306	313	320	327	334	341	348	355	362	369	376
71	136	143	150	157	165	172	179	186	193	200	208	215	222	229	236	243	250	257	265	272	279	286	293	301	308	315	322	329	338	343	351	358	365	372	379	386
72	140	147	154	162	169	177	184	191	199	206	213	221	228	235	242	250	258	265	272	279	287	294	302	309	316	324	331	338	346	353	361	368	375	383	390	397
73	144	151	159	166	174	182	189	197	204	212	219	227	235	242	250	257	265	272	280	288	295	302	310	318	325	333	340	348	355	363	371	378	386	393	401	408
74	148	155	163	171	179	186	194	202	210	218	225	233	241	249	256	264	272	280	287	295	303	311	319	326	334	342	350	358	365	373	381	389	396	404	412	420
75	152	160	168	176	184	192	200	208	216	224	232	240	248	256	264	272	279	287	295	303	311	319	327	335	343	351	359	367	375	383	391	399	407	415	423	431
76	156	164	172	180	189	197	205	213	221	230	238	246	254	263	271	279	287	295	304	312	320	328	336	344	353	361	369	377	385	394	402	410	418	426	435	443

Source: Courtesy of the National Heart, Lung, and Blood Institute.

Body Mass Index

In 1871 Dr. Quetelet developed the **Body Mass Index** (BMI), which has replaced body weight as the medical standard to define obesity. Although calculated using body height and weight, BMI provides a better evaluation of appropriate body weight than simple height-weight tables and correlates well with estimates of body fat obtained by underwater weighing.

Nevertheless, BMI does not provide a quantitative estimate of body fat and cannot distinguish between excess body fat and increased muscle in persons who weigh more than the standard. Stature influences body composition because taller people have greater bone mass, which adds to their body weight.

Thus, individuals with the same BMI may not have the same body composition. Despite these limitations, BMI is a useful tool relating the increase in health risk with excessive body weight, and providing a base line for intervention when more sophisticated equipment is not available.

$$BMI = Weight\ (kg) \div Height\ (m)^2$$

$$Weight: 1\ kg = 2.2\ lb$$

$$Height: 1\ m = 39.37\ inches$$

The desirable BMI range for adults is *18.5 to 24.9 kg/m²*. Health risks associated with overweight begin at *25 kg/m²* and become apparent at *30 kg/m²*. Values beyond *35 kg/m²* indicate severe obesity.

BMI is often used to evaluate the effects of overweight and obesity on morbidity and mortality. Age and gender become factors when evaluating the mortality risk associated with a rise in BMI, as older adults and women seem to better tolerate overweight or obesity than younger adults or men.

A recent analysis performed on 27 studies that followed up on nearly 3 million adults reported that overweight (*BMI = 25 to 29.9*) was associated with lower all-cause mortality rates, and persons with *a Grade 1 Obesity* (BMI = *30 to 34.9*) had similar mortality rates as those of desirable weight (*18.5 to 24.9 kg/m²*).

BMI measurements of *35* and over carried higher risk of death. These findings have raised questions as to whether all individuals with a BMI of *25* or higher should be approached about weight loss or if identification and intervention for other risk factors is a better approach

Abdominal Fat & Waist Circumference

Health and disease risk are influenced not only by the amount of body fat but also by where it is positioned. The pear shape, with a smaller waist and larger hip (gynoid shape), is characteristic of younger women and controlled to some extent by the female hormone estrogen.

The apple shape, with more fat around the abdomen (android shape), is common in men and postmenopausal women.

Because Abdominal (**Visceral**) Fat raises the Blood Lipid levels and increases the risk of Cardiovascular disease, extra weight around one's Middle is of greater harm than extra weight on the Hips or Thighs.

An appropriate Waist-to-Hip Ratio (WHR) is *0.9* or less for Men and *0.8* or less for Women.

These ratios indicate a smaller waist and a larger hip measurement.

Waist circumference has become a popular tool for evaluating abdominal fat and health status. The threshold for Abdominal Obesity as defined by waist circumference is greater

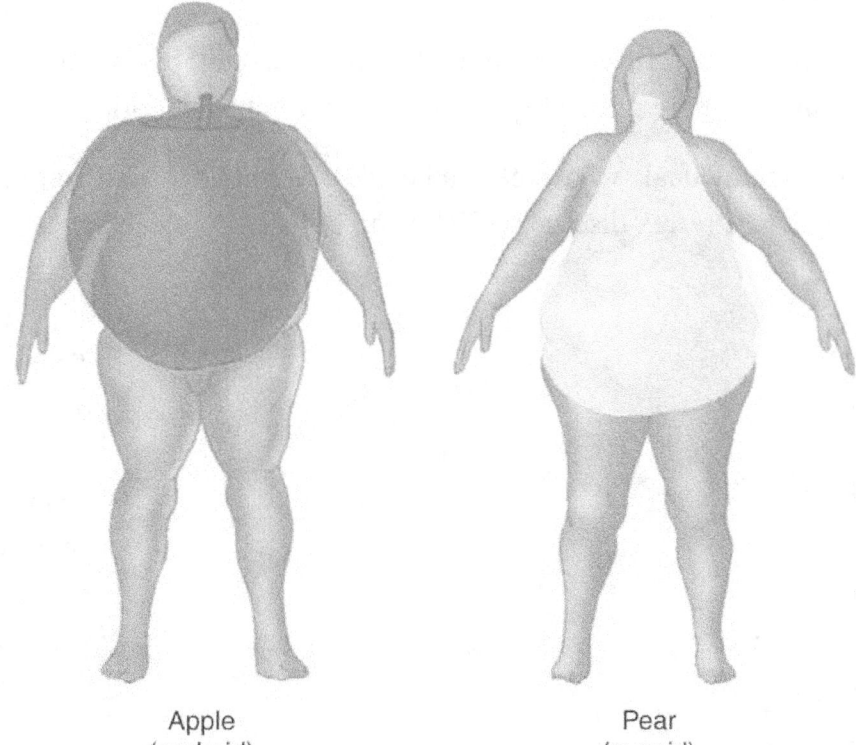

Apple
(android)

Pear
(gynoid)

than or equal to *88 cm* (35 inches) in Women and greater than or equal to *102 cm* (40 inches) in Men.

Fatness, Thinness & Health

Obesity & Health

Weight-related health problems can be divided into four categories: (1) *__Metabolic__*, (2) *__Degenerative__*, (3) *__Neoplastic__*, and (4) *__Anatomic__*.

• *__Metabolic__*: Type 2 diabetes, hypertension, elevated blood lipids, and the constellation of conditions associated with metabolic syndrome often accompany obesity. Regardless of total body fat, abdominal fat increases the risk of metabolic disorders.

• *__Degenerative__*: Obesity and physical disability are strongly linked. Osteoarthritis and joint problems, atherosclerotic changes, and pulmonary diseases are more serious in obese persons.

• *__Neoplastic__*: Many forms of cancer including colorectal, breast, prostate, esophageal, and ovarian cancer are more frequent in higher weight categories.

• *__Anatomic__*: Individuals who exceed a healthy weight have a greater risk of gastroesophageal reflux disease (GERD) and obstructive sleep apnea.

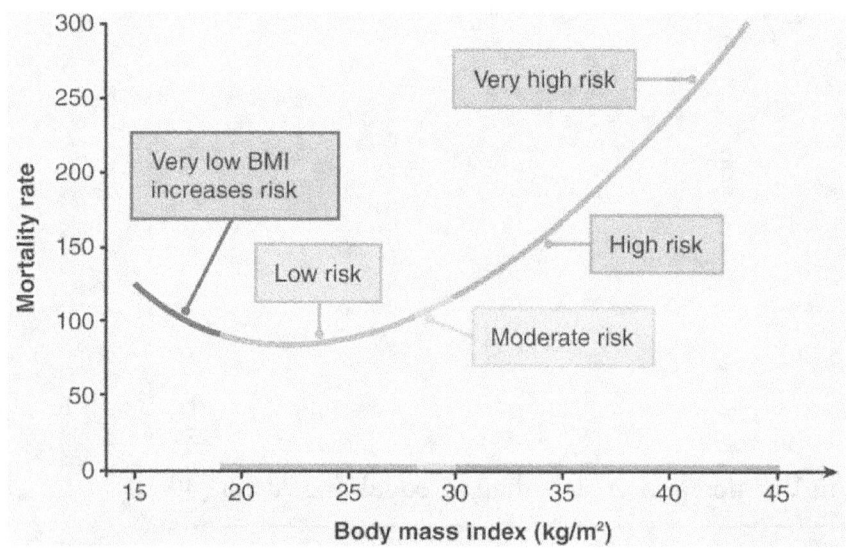

The current prevalence of Overweight and Obesity will increase health care costs in the years ahead. A 10-year follow-up of Medicare spending among normal weight, overweight, and obese older adults (classifications were based on BMI) indicated growing expenditures related to weight.

Obsession with Thinness

A trend opposite to obesity but equally harmful to health is the model of extreme thinness. Fueled by advertising dollars, an image of thinness drives the marketing of clothes, cosmetics, and food to teenagers and young adults.

Social pressures have created an abnormally thin and unrealistic ideal to the point that even fashion models express dissatisfaction with their overall body shapes.

Social discrimination against school-age children who are overweight can intensify the fear of weight gain.

Boys and girls as young as age 7 perceive their mothers' encouragement to remain thin, and develop restrained eating patterns and dissatisfaction with their bodies. When parents restrict food intake, children may react by overeating when those restricted foods are available outside the home.

Guilt feelings after eating certain foods and distorted perceptions of body size often form the basis for serious eating disorders that threaten nutritional and physical health. School programs, voluntary community programs, and sports programs that build self-esteem offer primary prevention for disordered eating.

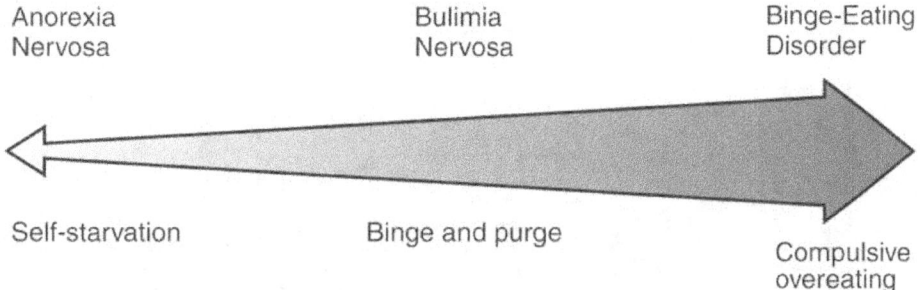

The ongoing quest for the perfect body has given rise to the chronic dieter who is constantly trying to restrict food intake. Although restrained eating is often seen in women, dieting is also a concern among boys and girls.

The family has a role in helping young people develop positive attitudes toward food.

Adolescents who reported positive communication and closeness within their families had more frequent meals with family and were less likely to follow inappropriate diets or engage in disordered eating behaviors.

Teens participating in weight-related sports are especially vulnerable to unhealthy weight-control practices, and preventive efforts should target parents and coaches.

Problem of Underweight

We have discussed the problem of excessive body weight and body fat, and situations in which individuals deliberately reduce their food intake. Now we consider the causes and effects of underweight caused by lack of food or debilitating illness.

Extreme underweight is associated with serious health problems in all age groups.

__Underweight__, defined as a BMI of Less than *18.5 kg/m²*, is relatively uncommon in the United States. A national survey identified only *2.2%* of adults as underweight, although a regional study found nearly *5%* of low-income children between the ages of 2 and 4 to be low weight for height.

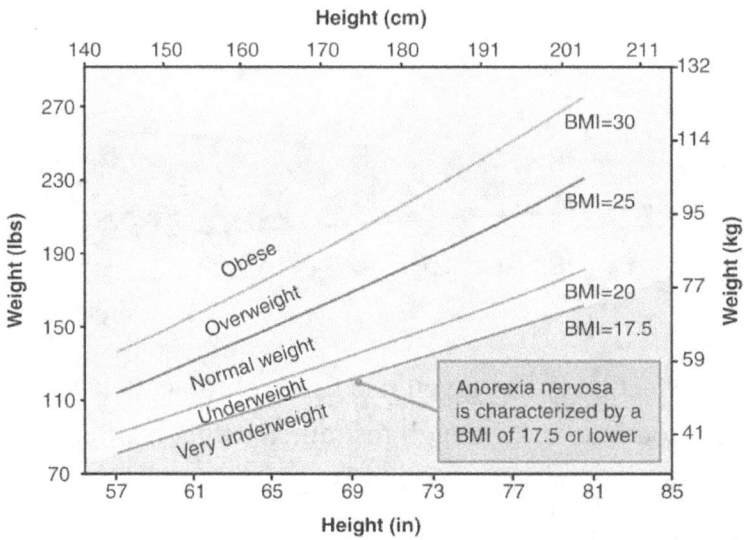

Low weight for age is associated with more than 2.2 million child deaths in developing countries, and those who do survive often experience long-term growth retardation and disability. Underweight springs from poverty, poor living conditions, long-term illness, or physiologic dysfunction. Infants, young children, and older adults are at greatest risk.

Resistance to infection is lower, general health is poorer, and physical strength is decreased in seriously underweight individuals.

Malnutrition and underweight stem from decreased food intake, increased energy requirements, or poor utilization of ingested nutrients.

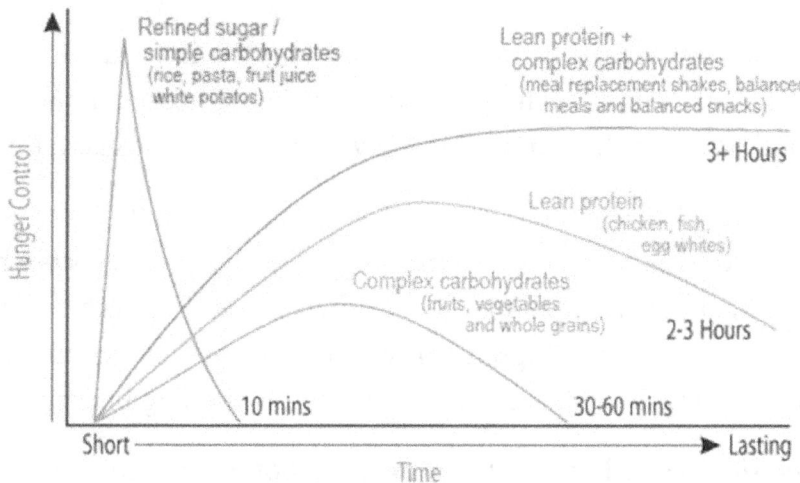

Nutritional Care

Underweight persons require special nutrition intervention to rebuild body tissues and nutrient stores. Food plans must be adapted to the individual's personal preferences, financial situation, and household concerns, and address any existing disease.

The dietary recommendation should be:

(1) High in Kcalories (at least 50% beyond standard needs);

(2) High in Protein to rebuild tissue;

(3) High in Carbohydrate to provide a primary energy source in an easily digested form;

(4) Moderate in Unsaturated Fats to add kcalories but not exceed recommended limits; and

(5) Optimum in Vitamins and Minerals, including supplements when deficiencies require them. A wide variety of food that is well seasoned and attractively presented helps revive a lagging appetite and the desire to eat. Meals and snacks spread throughout the day that include favorite foods increase interest in eating and promote optimal utilization of nutrients. Liquid nutritional supplements add kcalories and key nutrients. In extreme cases, tube feeding or *Total Parenteral Nutrition* (TPN) may be necessary.

• ***Poor food intake***: Lack of sufficient and appropriate food results in failure to thrive in children and older adults. Medications such as digoxin and chemotherapeutic agents contribute to the devastating weight loss known as ***Cachexia*** seen in cardiac failure and cancer.

Older people in poverty who live alone and lack transportation to a grocery store risk unwanted weight loss. Skilled nursing facilities are required to monitor body weight, as a patient's inability to self-feed can lead to significant weight loss. Self-imposed food restriction associated with eating disorders can result in life-threatening underweight.

• ***Increase in energy requirements***: Long-term **Hypermetabolic** conditions such as cancer, Acquired Immuno-Deficiency Syndrome (AIDS), advanced heart disease, or infection impose energy demands that drain the body's resources.

Hyperthyroidism increases caloric requirements. Extensive physical activity without a sufficient increase in energy intake will over time bring about inappropriate weight loss in the normal weight individual.

• ***Poor utilization of available nutrients***: Malabsorption associated with prolonged diarrhea, gastrointestinal disease, or laxative abuse depletes nutrient stores.

Cytokines produced by the immune system in response to chronic conditions such as cancer, chronic kidney disease, congestive heart failure, and AIDS accelerate the breakdown of body protein and fat.

Cytokines also interfere with the effective utilization of nutritional supplements, making it difficult to reverse the patient's deteriorating condition.

Estimated amounts of calories needed to maintain calorie balance for various gender and age groups at three different levels of physical activity. The estimates are rounded to the nearest 200 calories. An individual's calorie needs may be higher or lower than these average estimates.				
		Physical Activity Level[b]		
Gender	Age (years)	Sedentary	Moderately Active	Active
Child (female and male)	2–3	1,000–1,200[c]	1,000–1,400[c]	1,000–1,400[c]
Female[d]	4–8	1,200–1,400	1,400–1,600	1,400–1,800
	9–13	1,400–1,600	1,600–2,000	1,800–2,200
	14–18	1,800	2,000	2,400
	19–30	1,800–2,000	2,000–2,200	2,400
	31–50	1,800	2,000	2,200
	51 +	1,600	1,800	2,000–2,200
Male	4–8	1,200–1,400	1,400–1,600	1,600–2,000
	9–13	1,600–2,000	1,800–2,200	2,000–2,600
	14–18	2,000–2,400	2,400–2,800	2,800–3,200
	19–30	2,400–2,600	2,600–2,800	3,000
	31–50	2,200–2,400	2,400–2,600	2,800–3,000
	51 +	2,000–2,200	2,200–2,400	2,400–2,800

Energy Concerns with Low-Carb Diets

CARBOHYDRATES ARE OUR BODIES PREFERRED FORM OF ENERGY!!

The most extreme low-carb diet was pioneered by the late Robert Atkins, M.D. It promised a quick and long-lasting weight loss and prevention of chronic disease, all while allowing high-fat steak and bacon. Since then, other, more moderate low-carb diets have allowed small amounts of carb-rich foods, but they still cut out most grains as well as starchy vegetables and even fruit.

These diets have turned out to be less effective and less healthy than originally claimed. Often, the weight returned and as it did, problems such as high cholesterol and high blood pressure came back.

Low-carb diets usually begin with an "induction" phase that eliminates nearly every source of carbohydrate. Often, you'll consume as few as 20 grams of Carbs a day.

When Carb consumption falls *below* 100 grams, the body usually responds by burning Muscle Tissue for the Glycogen (stored Glucose) it contains.

When those Glycogen stores start to run out, the body resorts to burning Body Fat. But that is an *inefficient*, complicated way to produce Blood Sugar. The body tries to do it only when it *absolutely* has to (such as when it's starving)—and for a good reason.

Turning Fat into Blood Sugar comes at a price in the form of by-products called Ketones. They make your breath smell funny. They can also make you tired, lightheaded, headachy, and nauseated. Feeling lousy is certainly one way to dampen the appetite.

With virtually no carbs in your system, you may even have trouble concentrating. According to the Institute of Medicine of the National Academy of Sciences, the Human Brain requires the equivalent of 130 grams of Carbohydrates a day to function optimally—***and that is a minimum***.

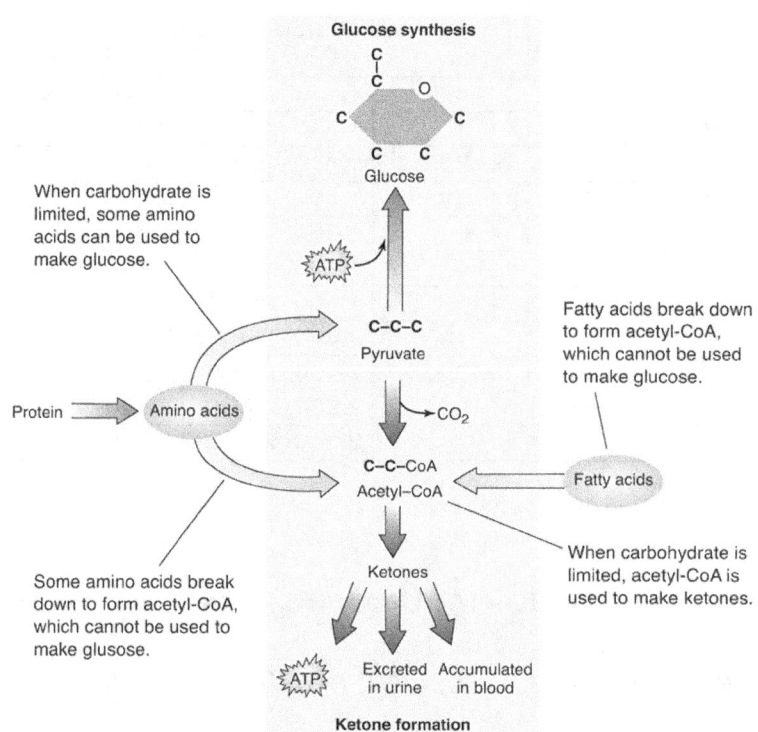

If you are overweight or obese and you have insulin resistance—and especially if you have prediabetes or diabetes—cutting way back on carbohydrates can have immediate health benefits.

Your Blood Sugar and insulin levels will go down, your Triglycerides and Blood Pressure may fall, and your levels of "good" HDL Cholesterol may rise.

But the low-carb diet will also wreak some havoc. When your body breaks down Lean Body Mass—muscle—for Energy, your metabolism slows because muscle tissue burns up a lot of calories.

This may be one reason that the weight often comes back after you have been avoiding Carbs for a while.

The alleged effects on your heart are also questionable. Especially if you switch to a high-saturated-fat diet, as people do when they start eating mainly steak and bacon, your "bad" LDL cholesterol will go up.

Levels of Homocysteine, an amino acid that increases the risk of heart disease, may also rise if you eat a lot of meat and too few vegetables.

And to get rid of the ketones produced when your body burns fat for energy, your kidneys need to work overtime, which raises your risk for kidney stones.

Ironically, low-carb diets may even interfere with insulin sensitivity; a certain amount of carbohydrate in your diet may be needed for the pancreas, which produces the insulin that keeps blood sugar in check, to work well.

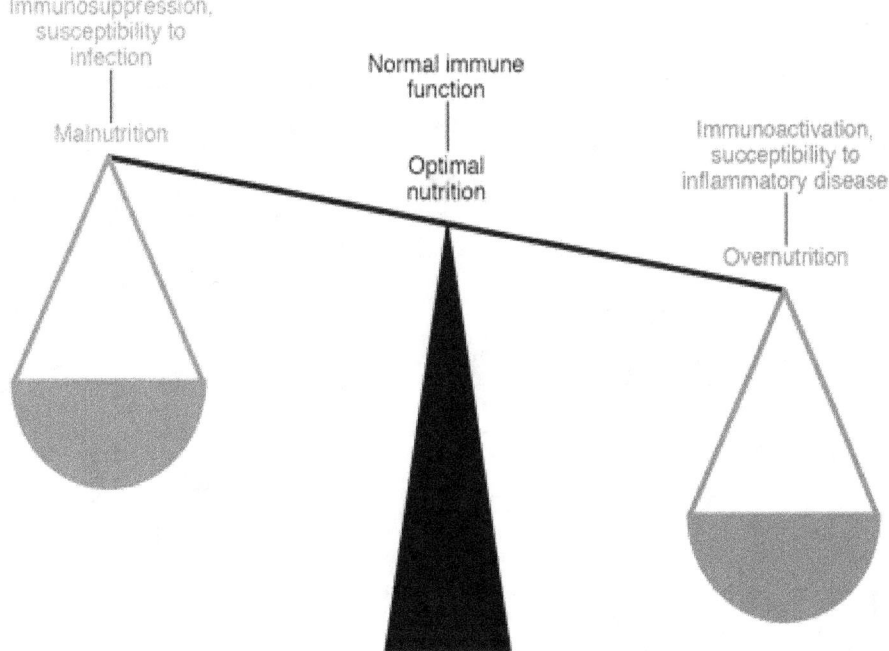

*Chapter Six ....

Energy & Work*

****

At this moment that you are reading these words, there are Trillions of Cells in your body hard at work turning the Chemical Energy of the food you ate yesterday into the Chemical Energy that will keep you alive today.

Energy in the atmosphere generates sweeping winds and powerful storms, while the ocean's energy drives mighty currents and incessant tides. Meanwhile, deep within Earth, Energy manifested in the form of Heat is moving the continent on which you are standing.

All situations where energy is expended have one thing in common. If you look at the event closely enough, you will find that, in accord with Newton's laws of motion, a force is being exerted on an object to make it move.

When your car burns gasoline, that fuel's Energy is what ultimately turns the wheels of your car, which then exert a Force on the road; the road exerts an Equal and Opposite Force on the car, pushing it forward.

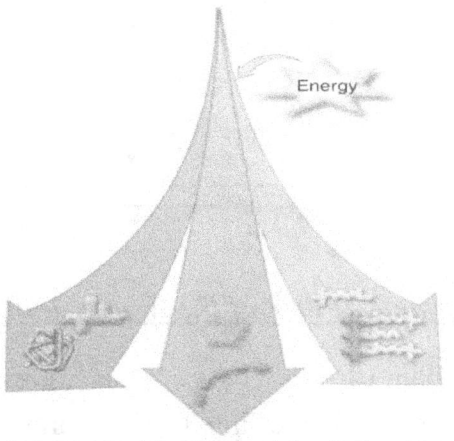

EXTRACTION OF ENERGY

Protein (amino acids)   Carbohydrates (sugars)   Fats (fatty acids)

Molecular building blocks

Energy

Amino acids and body protein   Glucose and glycogen   Fatty acids and lipids

BIOSYNTHESIS

When you climb the stairs, your Muscles exert a Force that lifts you upward against Gravity.

Even in the Cells of our bodies, a Force is exerted on our Molecules in Chemical Reactions which manifest Life.

Energy thus is intimately connected with the application of a Force.

In everyday conversation we may speak of someone having lots of energy, but in science the term Energy has a precise definition which is somewhat different from the ordinary conversational meaning. To see what us scientists mean when we talk about Energy, we must first intro- duce and elevate the familiar concept of *Work*.

Energy is what makes our Body go. There are several kinds of Energy that exist in our Biological systems: *Electrical Energy* in our Nerves and Muscles, *Chemical Energy* in the Synthesis of our Molecules, *Mechanical Energy* in the contraction of our Muscle, and *Thermal Energy* which is derived from all of these processes, that helps maintain our body Temperature.

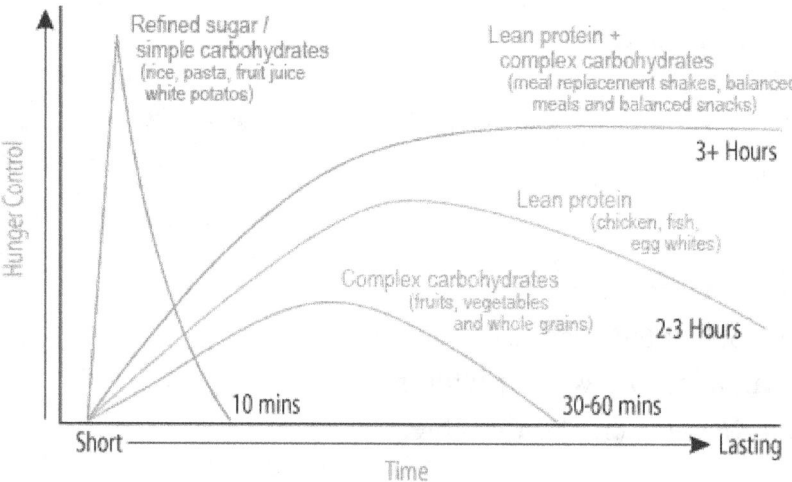

The Ultimate Source of the Energy found in our Biological Systems is the SUN.

The Radiant Life Energy from our Sun is absorbed by plants and used to convert simple Atoms and Molecules into Carbohydrates, Fats, and Proteins = Life Energy. The Life Energy of the Sun is transferred to within the Chemical Bonds of these food Molecules.

In order for our Cells to utilize this energy, they must break-down the foods in a manner that conserves most of the Energy contained within the bonds of the Carbohydrates, Fats, and Proteins of these foods.

Food is just a vehicle to for the un-seen Life Energy to be made manifest….the Life Energy is from the Sun….the Amount of Sun/Life Energy that was transformed in a particular food determines its Nutritional quality and value…..without the Life Energy from the Sun the plant is just an empty vehicle.

Page | 98

In addition, the final product of the breakdown must be a molecule the cell can use— Adenosine Tri-Phosphate (ATP).

Our Cells use ATP as the primary energy source for biological work, whether this work is electrical, mechanical, or chemical. In ATP, three phosphates are linked by high-energy bonds.

When a Chemical Bond between the Phosphates is broken, Energy is released and becomes available to be used by our Cells. At this point the ATP has been reduced to a lower Energy state, manifesting as *Adenosine Di-Phosphate* (ADP) and *Inorganic Phosphate* (P_i).

During our Muscular activity, ATP is constantly converted to ADP and P_i in order to make manifest the necessary Life Energy needed for successful completion of our Work. The ATP must be replaced as fast as it is used if our muscle is to continue to generate Force.

The muscle cell has a great capacity to replace ATP under a variety of work circumstances, from a short dash to a marathon.

	ENERGY SYSTEM*		
	Immediate	Nonoxidative	Oxidative
Duration of activity for which system predominates	0–10 seconds	10 seconds–2 minutes	>2 minutes
Intensity of activity for which system predominates	High	High	Low to moderately high
Rate of ATP production	Immediate, very rapid	Rapid	Slower but prolonged
Fuel	Adenosine triphosphate (ATP), creatine phosphate (CP)	Muscle stores of glycogen and glucose	Body stores of glycogen, glucose, fat, and protein
Oxygen used?	No	No	Yes
Sample activities	Weight lifting, picking up a bag of groceries	400-meter run, running up several flights of stairs	1500-meter run, 30-minute walk, standing in line for a long time

Edington and Edgerton devised a logical approach to help us understand how energy is supplied for muscle contraction—they divided the energy sources (ATP sources) into immediate, short term, and long term.

Good or proper Nutrition is essential to Performance, whether you are a marathon runner or a mall walker. Your diet must provide enough Life Energy to fuel activity, enough Protein to maintain muscle mass, sufficient Micro-Nutrients to metabolize the energy-yielding Nutrients, and enough Water to transport Nutrients and cool your body.

The major difference between the nutritional needs of a serious athlete and those of a casual exerciser is the amount of Energy and Water required.

Work

Scientists describe Work as performed whenever a Force is exerted over a Distance. Pick up this book and raise it a foot. Your muscles applied a Force Equal to the Weight (Gravitational Force/Pull) of the book over a distance of a foot = You did work.

This definition of work differs considerably from everyday usage. From a physicist's point of view, if you accidentally drive into a tree and smash your fender, Work has been done because a force deformed the car's metal a measurable distance.

On the other hand, a physicist would say that you haven't done any work if you spend an hour in a futile effort to move a large boulder, no matter how tired you get. Even though you have exerted a considerable force, the distance over which you exerted it is negligible.

Physicists provide an exact mathematical definition of their notion of Work.

In words:

 Work is equal to the force that is exerted times the distance over which it is exerted.

In equation form:

$$\underline{\textbf{\textit{W (Joules)}} = \textbf{\textit{Force (Newtons)}} \ \textbf{\textit{X}} \ \textbf{\textit{Distance (Meters)}}}$$

In symbols:

$$W = F \, X \, d$$

Energy

Energy is also defined as the Ability to do Work. If a system is capable of exerting a Force over a Distance, then that system possesses Energy. The amount of a system's Energy, which can be recorded in Joules or Foot-Pounds (the same units used for work), is a measure of how much Work the System might do. When a System runs out of Energy, it simply can't do any more Work = state of Death.

Power

Power provides a measure of both the Amount of Work done (or, equivalently, the amount of Energy Expended) and the Time it takes to do that Work. In order to complete a physical task quickly, you must generate more Power than if you do the same task slowly.

If you run up a flight of stairs, your Muscles need to generate more Power than they would if you walked up the same flight, even though you expend the same amount of Energy in either case. A power hitter in baseball swings the bat faster, converting the Chemical Energy in his muscles to Kinetic Energy more quickly than most other players.

Diet & Calories

The first Law of Thermodynamics has a great deal to say about the American obsession with weight and diet. Human beings take in Energy with our food and this Energy we usually measure in Kilocalories/KCals.

(Note that the Calorie we talk about in foods is defined as the Amount of Energy needed to raise the temperature of a Kilogram of Water by 1° Celsius = Kilocalorie.)

When a certain amount of energy is taken in, the first law says that only one of two things can happen to it: It can be Converted into Work and increased temperature of the surroundings, or it can be Stored.

If we take in more Energy than we expend, the excess is stored in Adipose Fat/Potential Energy. If, on the other hand, we take in less than we expend, energy must be removed from Storage/Adipose Fat to meet the deficit, and the amount of Body Fat DECREASES!!!

Here are a couple of rough rules you can use to calculate calories in your diet:

1. Under most circumstances, normal body maintenance uses up about 15 calories per day for each pound of body weight.

2. You must consume about 3,500 Kcals to gain a pound of Fat.

Suppose you weigh 150 pounds. **To keep your weight constant, you have to take in**:

$$\underline{\textit{150 pounds X 15 Kcals pound = 2,250 Kcals per day}}$$

If you wanted to lose one pound (3,500 Kcals) a week (7 days), you would have to reduce your daily Kcal intake by:

$$\frac{\underline{\textit{3500 calories}}}{\textit{7 days}} = \textit{500 calories per day}$$

Alternatively, the first Law says you can Increase your Energy use through exercise. Roughly speaking, to burn off 500 Kcals you would have to run 5 miles, bike 15 miles, or swim for an hour.

Energy Needs

The amount of energy expended for any activity depends on the intensity, duration, and frequency of the activity and the weight of the exerciser.

Whereas casual exercise may burn only 100 additional Kcals/day, the training required for an endurance athlete, such as a marathon runner, may increase Energy Expenditure by 2000 to 3000 Kcals/day.

Some athletes require 6000 Kcals/day to maintain their body weight. In general, the more intense the activity, the more energy it requires, and the more time spent exercising, the more energy is expended.

Running for 60 minutes, for instance, involves more work than walking for the same amount of time and therefore requires more energy.

Immediate Sources of Energy

The very limited amount of ATP stored in a muscle might meet the energy demands of a maximal effort lasting about 1 sec.

Phosphocreatine (PC), another High-Energy Phosphate Molecule that is stored in our Muscle, is the most important immediate source of Energy.

PC can donate its Phosphate Molecule (and the energy therein) to ADP in order to make ATP, allowing our muscle to continue producing Force.

$$PC + ADP \rightarrow ATP + C$$

This reaction takes place as fast as our Muscle forms ADP. Unfortunately, the PC store in our Muscle can manifest only 3 to 5 Seconds when our muscle is working maximally. This process does not require Oxygen and is one of the **Anaerobic Energy** (without oxygen) mechanisms for producing ATP.

PC is the primary source of ATP during a shot put, a vertical jump, or the first seconds of a sprint.

Short-Term Sources of Energy

As our Muscle's store of PC decreases, the Fiber of our Muscle breaks down Glucose (a Simple Sugar) to produce ATP at a high rate. This Glucose is obtained from our Blood or our Muscle's Glycogen store.

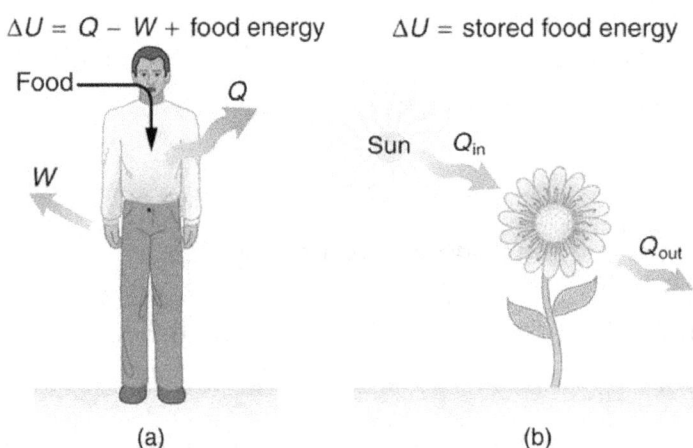

The multienzyme pathway for Glucose metabolism is called **Glycolysis**, and it does not require Oxygen to function (like the break-down of PC, it too is an Anaerobic process).

Glucose → 2 Pyruvic Acid + 2 ATP

In Glycolysis, Glucose is broken down into two molecules of Pyruvic Acid; in the process, ADP is converted to ATP, allowing our muscle to maintain a high rate of Work. But Glycolysis can only continue for a limited time.

When Glycolysis operates at high speed, Pyruvic Acid is converted to Lactic Acid, and this Lactic Acid (Lactate) accumulates in our Muscle and the Blood.

This accumulation of Lactic Acid in the muscle impedes the rate of Glycogen metabolism and may interfere with the mechanism involved in Muscle contraction.

Supplying ATP via Glycolysis has its shortcomings, but it does allow a person to run at Fast speeds for Short distances. This Short-Term Energy source is of primary importance in events involving maximal work lasting about 2 min.

ATP and Energy

- Releasing Energy
  - Energy stored in ATP is released by breaking the chemical bond between the second and third phosphates.

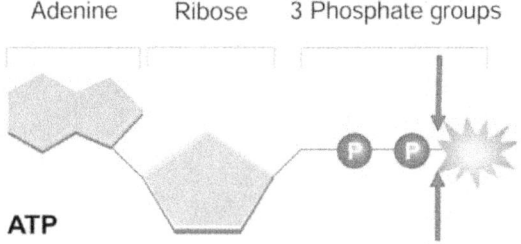

Adenine   Ribose   3 Phosphate groups

ATP

Long-Term Sources of Energy

Long-term sources of our Energy involve the production of ATP from a variety of fuels, but this method also requires the utilization of Oxygen—in other words, it is **Aerobic Energy**. The primary fuels include Muscle Glycogen, Blood Glucose, Plasma free fatty acids, and Intra-Muscular Fats.

Protein provides only a Small percentage of Energy for Muscle contraction, so the focus is on Carbs and Fat. Glucose is broken down in Glycolysis (as described previously), but in this case the Pyruvic Acid is taken into the **Mitochondria** of our Cell, where it is converted to a 2-Carbon fragment (Acetyl CoA) that enters the Krebs cycle.

Fats are taken into our Mitochondria, where they are also broken down into Acetyl CoA, which again enters the Krebs cycle.

The energy originally contained in the Glucose and fats is extracted from the Acetyl CoA and is used to generate ATP in the Electron transport chain in a process called *Oxidative Phosphorylation*, which requires Oxygen.

Carbohydrate and fat + O₂ → ATP

$$\textit{Carbohydrate and fat} + O_2 \rightarrow ATP$$

ATP production via aerobic mechanisms is slower than production from immediate and short-term sources of energy, and during submaximal work it may be 2 or 3 min before the ATP needs of the cell are met completely by this aerobic process.

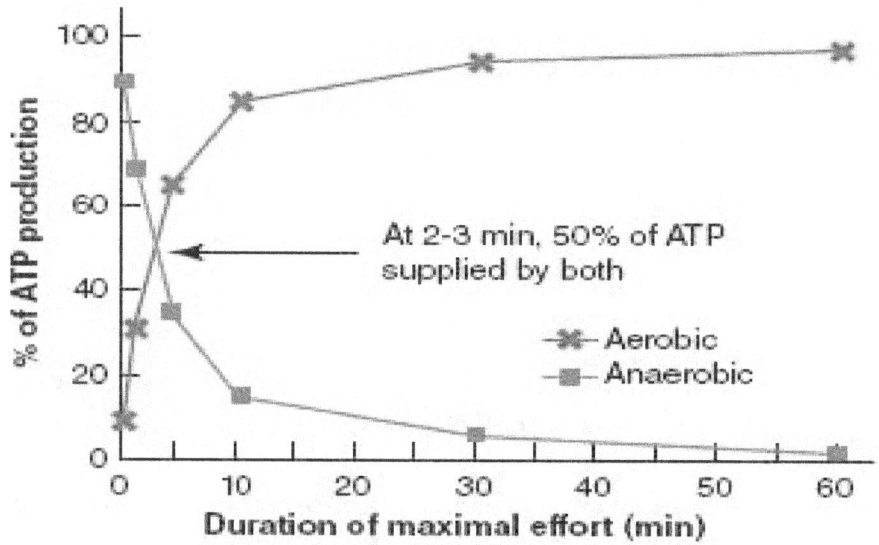

One reason for this lag is the time it takes for the Heart to increase the delivery of Oxygen-enriched Blood to the Muscles at the rate needed to meet the ATP demands of the Muscle.

Another is the time it takes for Oxidative Phosphorylation to increase its rate of ATP production from resting levels to that needed to meet the exercise demand.

Aerobic production of ATP is the primary means of supplying energy to the muscle in maximal work lasting more than 2 minutes and in all sub-maximal work.

Interaction of Exercise Intensity, Exercise Duration & Energy Production

The proportion of energy coming from anaerobic sources (immediate and short-term energy) is influenced by the intensity and duration of the activity. During an all-out activity lasting less than 1 min (e.g., a 400 m dash), the muscles obtain most of their ATP from anaerobic sources.

In a 2 to 3 min maximal effort, approximately 50% of the energy comes from anaerobic sources and 50% comes from aerobic sources; in a 10 min maximal effort, the anaerobic component drops to 15%.

For a 30 min all-out effort, the anaerobic component is about 5%, and it is even smaller in a typical submaximal 30 min training session.

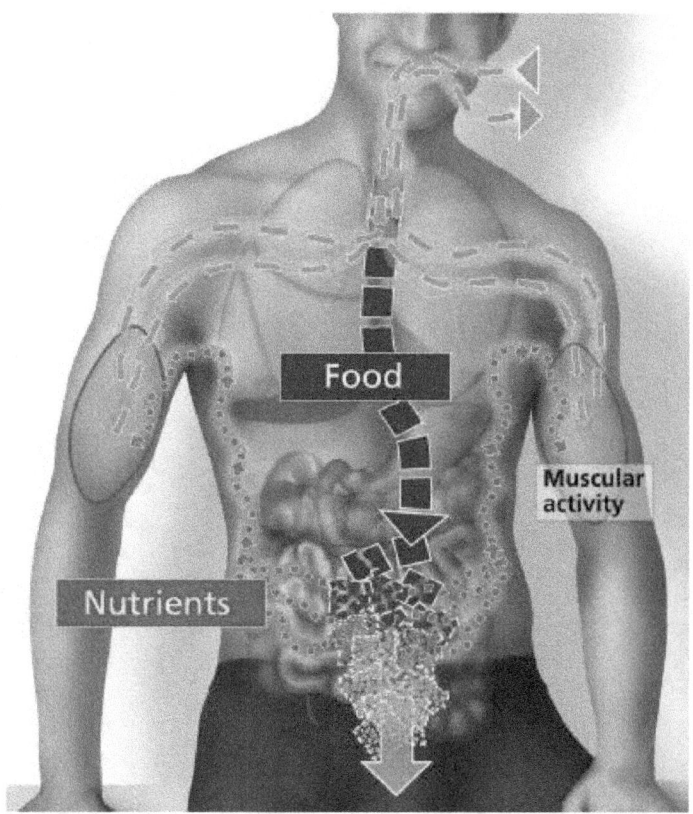

Page | 109

Chapter Seven .... Life Energy & Trophic Levels

****

All of Earth's systems, both living and nonliving, transforms the Radiant Life Energy of the Sun into other forms. Just how much Energy is available, and how is it used by living organisms is the catalyst for Abundant Life.

At the top of our Earth's Atmosphere, the incoming energy of the Sun is **1,400 Watts per Square Meter**. To calculate the Total Energy of this Solar Power, we first need to calculate Earth's cross-sectional area in Square Meters. The Earth's radius is 6,375 kilometers (6,375,000 meters), and so the cross-sectional area is

$$\text{area of a circle} = \text{pi} \times (\text{radius})^2$$
$$= 3.14 \times (6,375,000 \text{ m})^2$$
$$= 1.28 \times 10^{14} \text{ m}^2$$

Thus, the total power received at the top of Earth's atmosphere is

$$\text{power} = \text{solar energy per m}^2 \times \text{Earth's cross-sectional area}$$
$$= 1,400 \text{ watts/m}^2 \times 1.28 \times 10^{14} \text{ m}^2$$
$$= 1.79 \times 10^{17} \text{ watts}$$

Each second, the top of Earth's atmosphere receives **1.79×10^{17}** Joules of Energy, but fortunately for us, that is more than twice the amount that actually reaches the surface. When Solar Radiation encounters the top of the Atmosphere, about 25% of it is immediately reflected back out into space.

Another 25% is absorbed by Gases in our Atmosphere, and Earth's surface reflects an additional 5% back into Space.

These processes leave about 45% of the initial amount to be absorbed at Earth's surface.

All living systems take their Energy from this 45% but absorb only a small portion of this amount—only about 4% to run Photosynthesis and supply our entire food chain. A much larger portion heats the ground or air, or evaporates water from lakes, rivers, and oceans.

This makes the concept of Growing our own Food make even more sense and should stress a sense of urgency in those that haven't already began a Garden to do so IMMEDIATELY!!!

The concept of the Food Chain and its trophic levels is particularly useful when tracking the many changes of Energy as it flows through living systems of Earth.

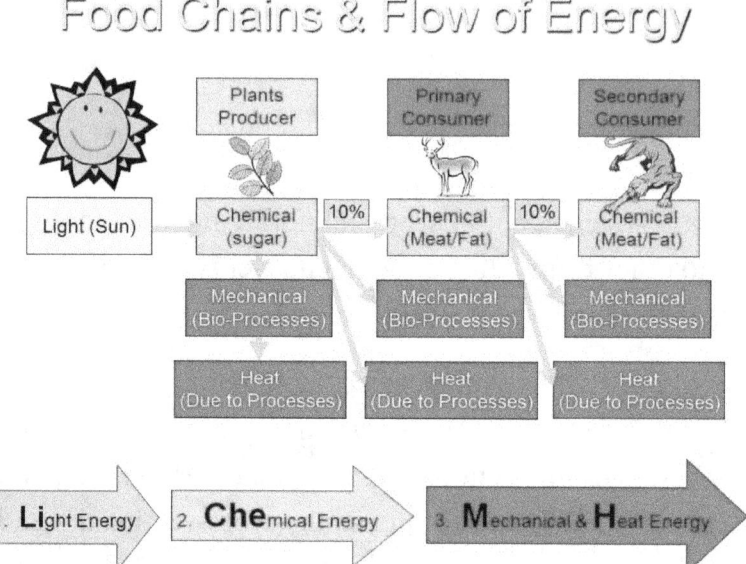

A trophic level consists of all organisms that get their energy from the same source.

In this ranking scheme, all plants that make manifest Life Energy from Photosynthesis are in the First Trophic level.

These plants all absorb the un-seen Life Energy from our Sun and use it to make manifest Seen Chemical Reactions that in-turn makes the plant Tissues and other Complex Molecules subsequently available to be used as Life Energy sources.

The Second Trophic level includes all Herbivores = HUMANS and other animals that get our Life Energy by eating plants of the first trophic level. We share this level with other animals like cows, rabbits, and many insects.

By growing our own food, we create a Straight Line to our ONLY source of Life Energy = the Sun. We ensure that we get Quality and Life Energy Dense food = Successfully Building and Maintaining our own Supreme Health and Fitness!

The Third Trophic level, as you might expect, consists of Carnivores—animals that get their energy by eating organisms in the Second Trophic level.

This third level includes such familiar animals as wolves, eagles, and lions, as well as insect-eating birds, blood-sucking ticks and mosquitoes, and many other organisms.

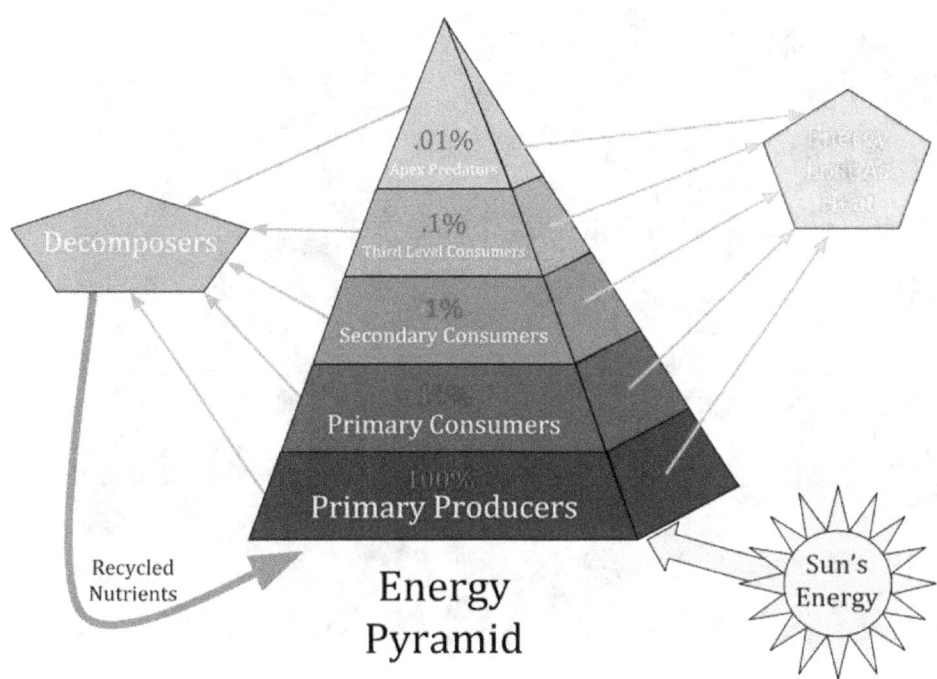

A few more groups of organisms fill out the scheme of Trophic levels on Earth. Carnivores that eat other carnivores, such as killer whales, occupy the Fourth Trophic level. Termites, vultures, and a host of bacteria and fungi get their energy from feeding on dead organisms and are generally placed in a trophic level separate from the four we have just described.

The usual conventional science is that this trophic level is not given a number because the dead organisms can come from any of the other trophic levels.

Although you might expect it to be otherwise, the efficiency with which solar energy is used by Earth's organisms is very low, despite the struggle by all these organisms to use energy efficiently.

When Sunlight falls, for example, on a cornfield in the middle of Iowa in August—arguably one of the best situations in the world for plant growth—only a small percentage of the solar energy striking the field is actually transformed as Chemical Energy in the plants.

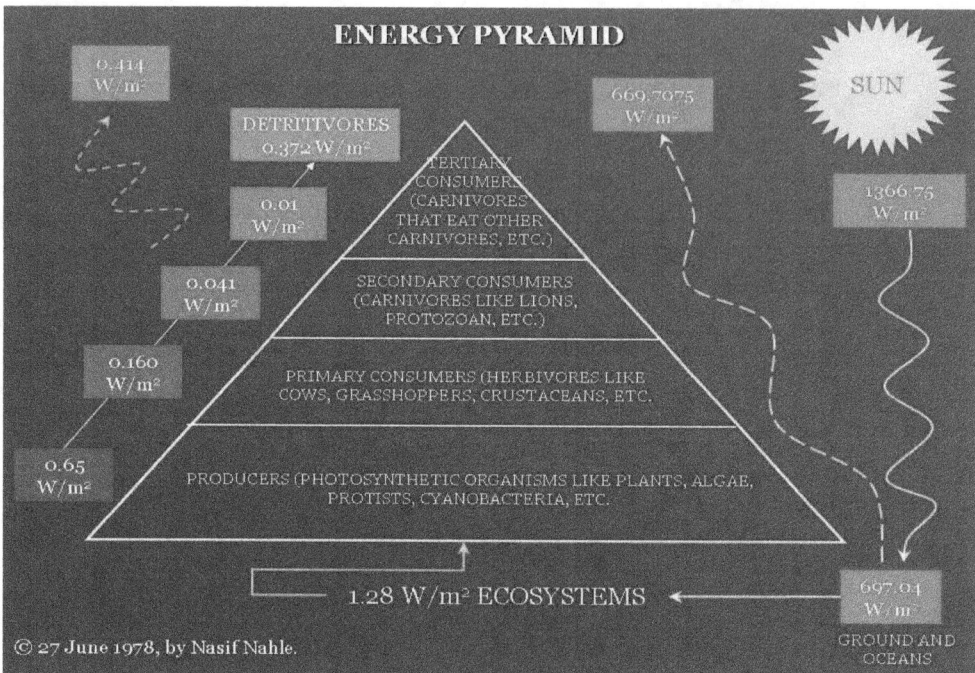

All the rest of the Energy is reflected, Heats up the soil, evaporates Water, or performs some other function.

It is a general rule that no plants anywhere transform as much as 10% of Solar/Life Energy available to them.

The same situation applies to trophic levels above the first. Typically, less than 10% of a plant's Chemical Potential Energy is made manifest as tissue in the animal of the Second Trophic level that eats the Plants.

That is, less than about 1% (10% of 10%) of the original Life Energy in the Sunlight is transformed into Chemical Energy of the Second Trophic level.

Continuing with the same pattern, animals in the Third Trophic level also use less than 10% of the Energy available from the second level.

Carbohydrate, Fat & Protein Needs

The Source of Energy in a person with an Active lifestyle can be just as important as the Amount. To maximize Glycogen stores and optimize performance, a diet providing about 6 to 10 Grams of Carbohydrate/kg of Body Weight per day is recommended for athletes in training.

The recommended amount of Fat is the same as that for the general population—between 20 and 35% of Energy. To allow for enough Carbs and Fat intakes at the lower end of this range may be needed for some athletes.

Diets that are very low in Fat (less than 20% of calories) do not benefit performance.

Protein is NOT a significant Energy source, accounting for only about 5% of Energy expended, but dietary Protein is needed to maintain and repair Lean Tissues, including Muscle.

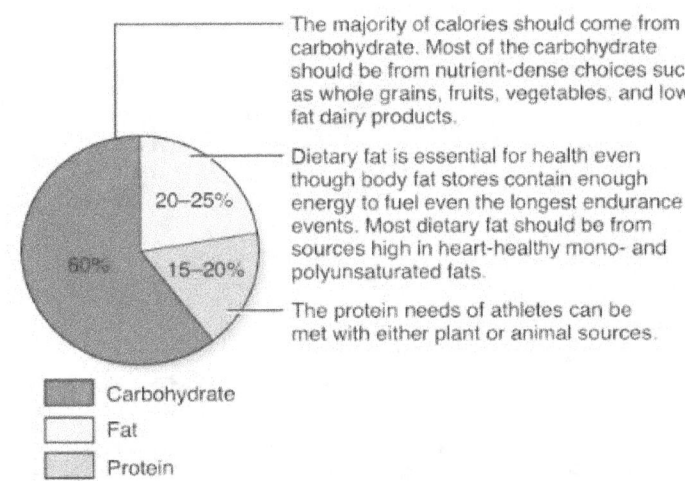

The majority of calories should come from carbohydrate. Most of the carbohydrate should be from nutrient-dense choices such as whole grains, fruits, vegetables, and low-fat dairy products.

Dietary fat is essential for health even though body fat stores contain enough energy to fuel even the longest endurance events. Most dietary fat should be from sources high in heart-healthy mono- and polyunsaturated fats.

The protein needs of athletes can be met with either plant or animal sources.

Carbohydrate

Fat

Protein

A diet in which 15 to 20% of calories come from Protein will meet the needs of most athletes.

The proportions of Carbs, Fat, and Protein recommended in the diets of athletes, shown in the pie chart above are within the ranges recommended for the general population: 45 to 65% of total Energy from Carbohydrate, 20 to 35% of Energy from Fat, and 10 to 35% of Energy from Protein.

Antioxidants & Oxidative damage

Exercise increases the amount of Oxygen used by the Muscles and significantly increases the rate of ATP-producing Metabolic Reactions. This increased Oxygen intake and use increases the production of Free-radicals, which can lead to or cause Oxidative damage and contribute to Muscle Fatigue.

To protect the body from this oxidative damage, our muscle cells contain antioxidant defenses, some of which may interact with dietary Antioxidants such as vitamin C, Vitamin E, β-Carotene, and Selenium.

Despite the importance of antioxidants for health and performance, there is little evidence that supplementation with antioxidants improves human performance.

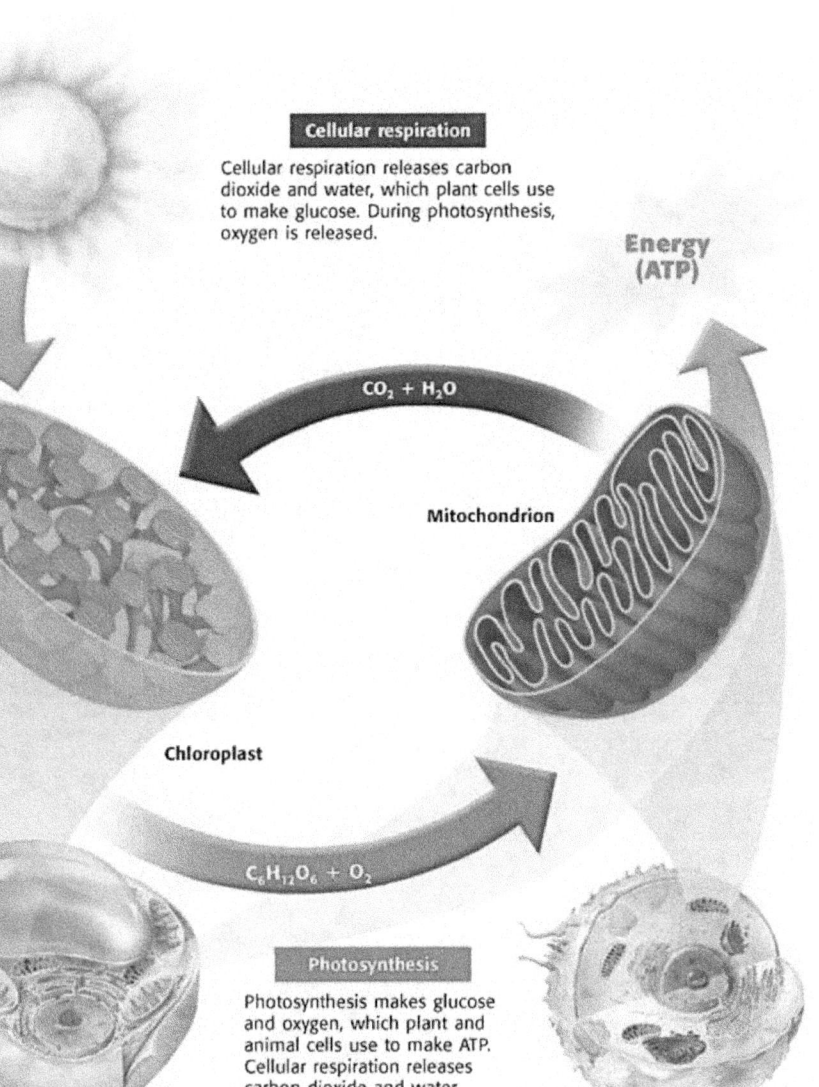

Cellular respiration

Cellular respiration releases carbon dioxide and water, which plant cells use to make glucose. During photosynthesis, oxygen is released.

Energy (ATP)

Light energy

$CO_2 + H_2O$

Mitochondrion

Chloroplast

$C_6H_{12}O_6 + O_2$

Photosynthesis

Photosynthesis makes glucose and oxygen, which plant and animal cells use to make ATP. Cellular respiration releases carbon dioxide and water.

Plant cell

Animal cell

*Chapter Eight ...

Muscle Structure & Function *

****

Exercise translates into Movement, and Movement requires Muscle Action. When we discuss our Human Physiology related to Exercise and Endurance Training, we must start with our Skeletal Muscle, the Tissue that converts the Chemical Energy of ATP to Mechanical Work.

Our bodies are NOT created to continuously Exercise for long durations, any routine/regimen longer than 30 mins significantly increases our chances for damage while simultaneously decreasing our ability to Build or Maintain our Supreme Health and Fitness.

Being Over-Weight is caused from Fat or MUSCLE. ....THE HEALTH ISSUES ARE THE SAME!!!!

How does a muscle do this?

The following picture shows the structure of Skeletal Muscle, from the intact Muscle to the smallest functional unit within the Muscle.

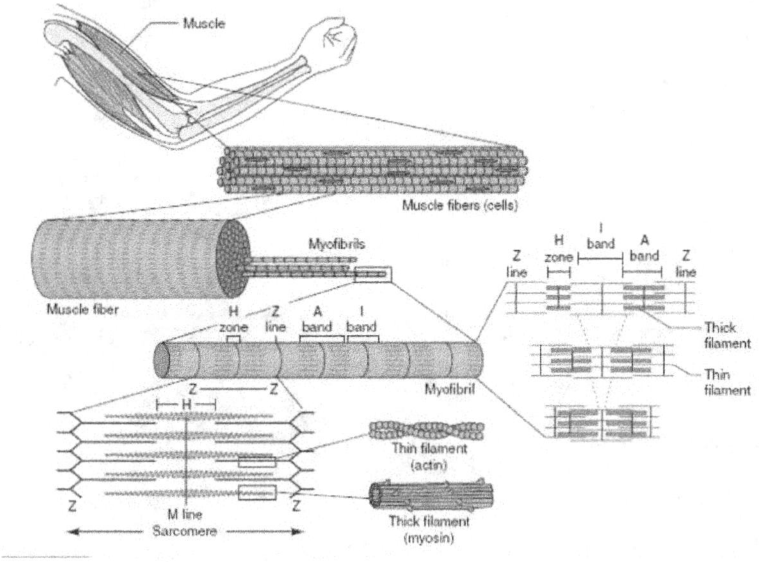

A **Muscle Fiber** is a Cylindrical Cell that has repeating light and dark bands, giving it the name **Striated Muscle**.

The Striations are attributable to a more basic structural component called the **Myofibril,** which runs the length of the Muscle.

Each Myofibril is composed of a long series of **Sarcomeres,** the fundamental units of Muscle Contraction. The associated figure shows that the Sarcomere contains the thick *Page / 119* filament **Myosin** and the thin filament **Actin** and is bounded by Connective Tissue called the **Z Line**.

An enlargement of two Sarcomeres in the above figure shows that the **A Band, I Band,** and **H Zone** and the changes that take place when the Sarcomere moves from the resting state to the contracted state. The I Band is composed of actin and is bisected by the Z Line, and the A Band is composed of Myosin and Actin.

According to the **Sliding-Filament Theory** used to describe Muscle Contraction, the thin Actin Filaments slide over the thick Myosin Filaments, pulling the Z Lines toward the center of the Sarcomere. According to this model, the entire Muscle shortens, but the Contractile Proteins do not change size.

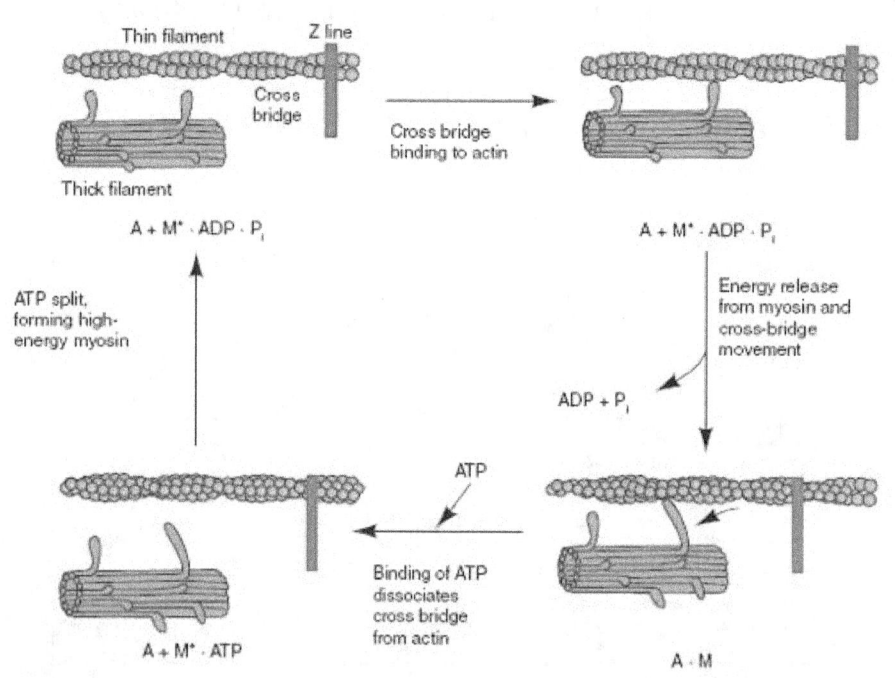

So how does the muscle release the energy in ATP for shortening?

If ATP is the energy supply, then an ATPase (an Enzyme) must exist in muscle to split ATP and release the Potential Energy contained within its Bonds.

ATPase is found in an extension of the thick Myosin Filament, the **Cross-bridge**, which also can bind to actin. The following figure shows how ATP, the Cross-bridge, and actin interact to shorten the Sarcomere.

At rest, two Proteins that are associated with Actin block the interaction of Myosin with Actin: **Troponin**, which has the capacity to bind Calcium, and **Tropomyosin**. When a Muscle is depolarized (excited) by a Motor Nerve, the action potential spreads over the surface of the Muscle Fiber and enters the fiber through special channels called **Transverse Tubules** (this process is step 1 in the figure).

Once inside the muscle fiber, this wave of depolarization spreads over the **Sarcoplasmic Reticulum (SR)**, a membrane that surrounds the Myofibril, and the SR releases Calcium (Ca^{2+}) into the Sarcoplasm (step 2 in the figure).

When this Calcium binds with Troponin, the Tropomyosin aligns the Cross-bridge binding site on the actin so that the Myosin cross-bridge can interact with it (step 3 in the figure).

When the Cross-bridge binds to actin, energy is released, the Cross-bridge moves, and the Sarcomere shortens (step 4 in the figure).

This sequence repeats as long as there is Calcium is present and the muscle can replace the ATP it uses.

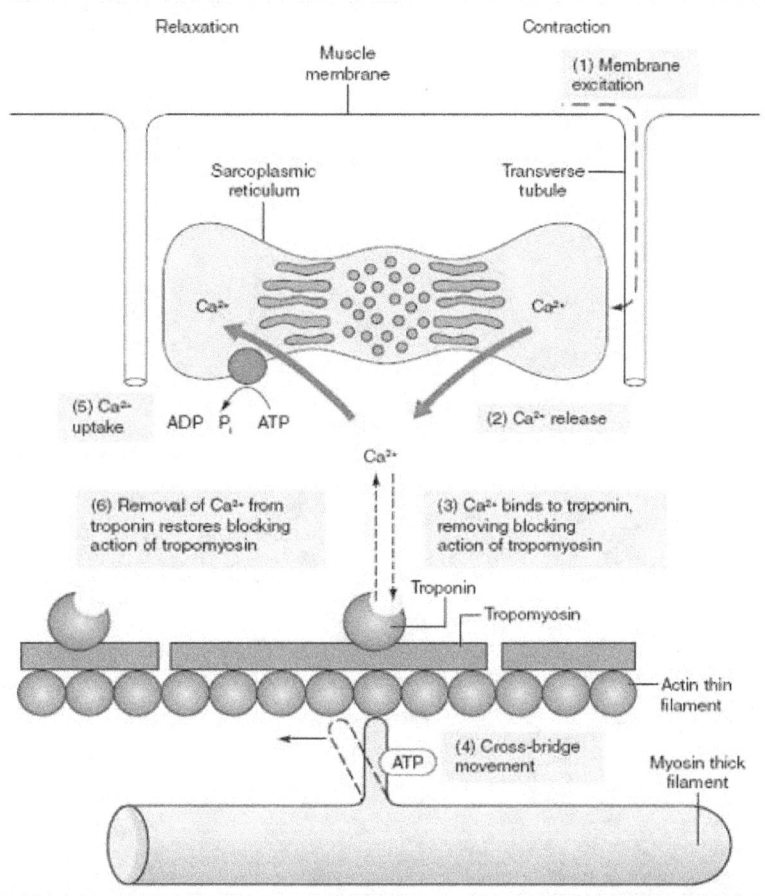

Understanding Our Human Energy System!

The muscle relaxes when the Calcium is pumped back into the SR and Troponin and Tropomyosin can again block the interaction of Actin and Myosin (steps 5 and 6 in the figure).

The Muscle needs ATP for moving the Cross-bridge, pumping the Calcium back to the SR, and maintaining the resting membrane potential that allows the Muscle to be depolarized.

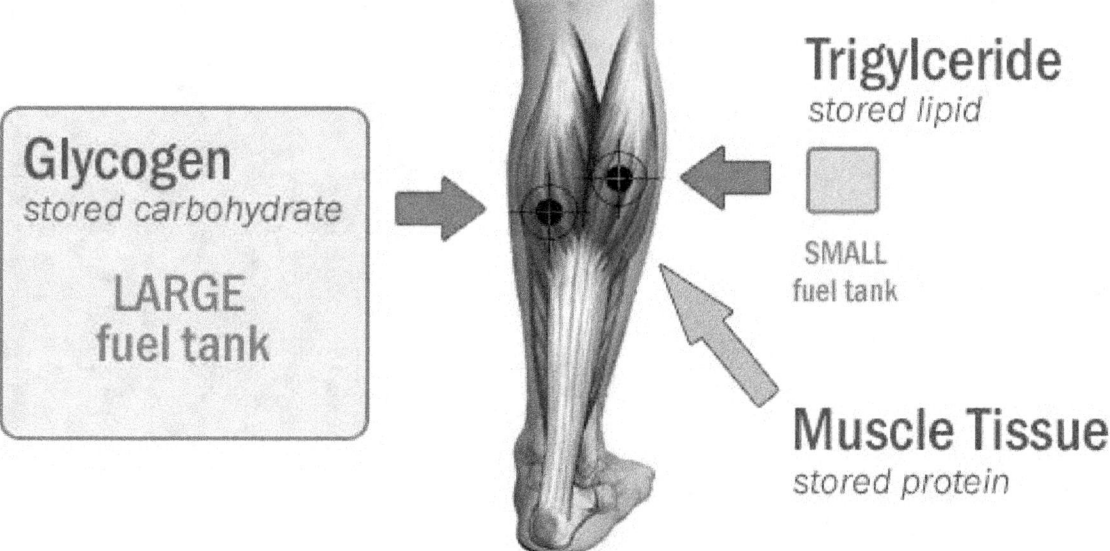

*Chapter Nine ....

Fuel Utilization During Exercise*

****

In general, protein contributes less than 5% to total energy production during exercise, and for the purpose of our discussion of Understanding Human Energy, it will be ignored. Ignoring Protein leaves Carbohydrate (Muscle Glycogen and Blood Glucose, which is derived from Liver Glycogen) and Fat (Adipose Tissue and Intramuscular Fat) as the primary fuels for exercise…..as it should be.

The ability of R to provide good information about the metabolism of fat and Carbohydrate during exercise stems from the following observations about the metabolism of Fat and Glucose.

Respiratory Quotients for Carbohydrate and Fat

For glucose ($C_6H_{12}O_6$),

$$C_6H_{12}O_6 + 6\,O_2 \rightarrow 6\,CO_2 + 6\,H_2O + energy$$

$$R = \frac{6\,CO_2}{6\,O_2} = 1.0.$$

For palmitate ($C_{16}H_{32}O_2$, a fatty acid),

$$C_{16}H_{32}O_2 + 23\,O_2 \rightarrow 16\,CO_2 + 16\,H_2O + energy$$

$$R = \frac{16\,CO_2}{23\,O_2} = 0.7.$$

When $R = 1.0$, 100% of the Energy is derived from Carbohydrate, 0% from Fat; when $R = 0.7$, the *reverse* is true.

When $R = 0.85$, approximately 50% of the Energy comes from Carbohydrate and 50% comes from Fat.

For the R measurement to be correct, the subject must be in a steady state. If Lactic Acid is increasing in the Blood, the Plasma Bicarbonate (HCO_3^-) buffer store reacts with the Acid (H^+) and produces CO_2, which must be *exhaled* so that the exerciser is stimulated to Hyperventilate:

$$H^+ + HCO_3^- \rightarrow H_2CO_3 \rightarrow H_2O + CO_2.$$

This CO_2 does not come from the Aerobic metabolism of Carbohydrate and Fat, so when it is exhaled, it results in an *overestimation* of the true value of R. During strenuous work, Lactic Acid is produced in great amounts, and R can exceed 1.0.

Effect of Exercise Intensity on Fuel Utilization

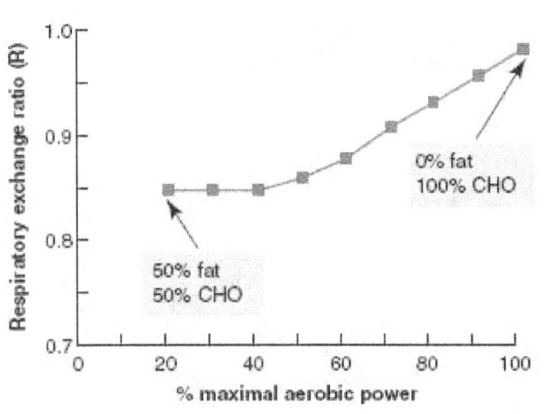

The following figure shows how R changes during progressive work up to VO_2max. In the progressive test, R increases at about 40% to 50% VO_2max, indicating that type II(a) Fibers are being recruited and Carbohydrate (CHO) is becoming a more important fuel source. Using Carbs provides an adaptive advantage—the Muscle obtains about 6% *more* Energy from each liter of O_2 when Carbs are used (5 kcal $\cdot$ L^{-1}) *compared* with when Fat is used (4.7 kcal $\cdot$ L^{-1}).

Carbohydrate fuels for muscular exercise include Muscle Glycogen and Liver Glycogen, which maintains the Blood Glucose concentration. Muscle Glycogen is the primary Carb fuel for heavy exercise lasting less than 2 hr, and inadequate Muscle Glycogen results in premature fatigue.

As Muscle Glycogen is depleted during prolonged heavy exercise, Blood Glucose becomes more important in supplying the Carbohydrate fuel.

Toward the end of heavy exercise lasting 3hrs or more, your Blood Glucose provides almost all the Carb used by the Muscles. Therefore, heavy exercise is limited by the availability of Carbohydrate fuels, which must be either stored in abundance before exercise (Muscle Glycogen) or replaced through the ingestion of Carbs during exercise (Blood Glucose).

Effect of Exercise Duration on Fuel Utilization

R changes during a 90 min test performed at 65% of the subject's VO_2max. R decreases over time, indicating a greater reliance on Fat as a fuel.

The Fat is derived from both Intramuscular Fat stores and Adipose Tissue, which releases free Fatty Acids into the Blood to be carried to the Muscle for use as Energy. Using more Fat spares the remaining Carb stores and extends the time to exhaustion.

Effect of Diet and Training on Fuel Utilization

The type of fuel used during exercise depends on diet. It has been demonstrated clearly that a diet high in carbohydrate (versus an average diet) increases the muscle glycogen content and extends the time to exhaustion.

Further, the muscle gains a greater capacity to increase its Glycogen store if a person performs strenuous exercise before eating high-carb meals.

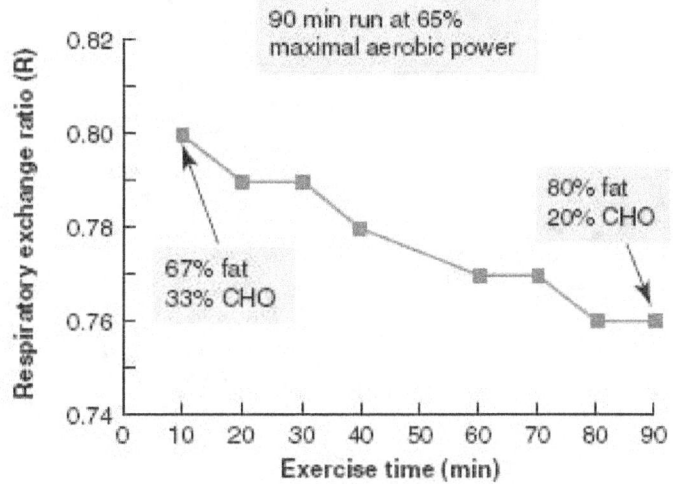

Finally, during prolonged heavy exercise, Carb drinks help to maintain the Blood Glucose concentration and extend the time to fatigue.

Endurance training increases the number of Mitochondria in the Muscles involved in the training program.

Having more Mitochondria increases the ability of the Muscle to use Fat as a fuel and to process the available Carbohydrates Aerobically.

This ability spares the Carbohydrate store and reduces lactate production, both of which favorably and significantly influences performance.

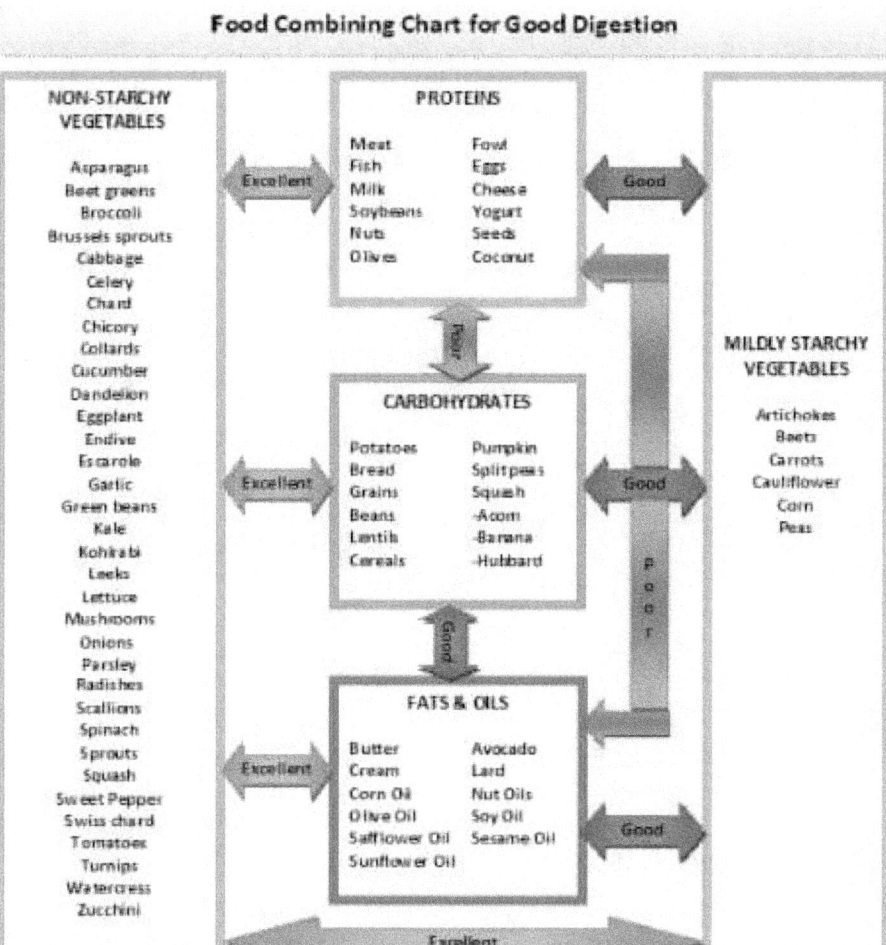

Food Combining Chart for Good Digestion

NON-STARCHY VEGETABLES

Asparagus
Beet greens
Broccoli
Brussels sprouts
Cabbage
Celery
Chard
Chicory
Collards
Cucumber
Dandelion
Eggplant
Endive
Escarole
Garlic
Green beans
Kale
Kohlrabi
Leeks
Lettuce
Mushrooms
Onions
Parsley
Radishes
Scallions
Spinach
Sprouts
Squash
Sweet Pepper
Swiss chard
Tomatoes
Turnips
Watercress
Zucchini

PROTEINS

Meat   Fowl
Fish   Eggs
Milk   Cheese
Soybeans   Yogurt
Nuts   Seeds
Olives   Coconut

CARBOHYDRATES

Potatoes   Pumpkin
Bread   Split peas
Grains   Squash
Beans   -Acorn
Lentils   -Banana
Cereals   -Hubbard

FATS & OILS

Butter   Avocado
Cream   Lard
Corn Oil   Nut Oils
Olive Oil   Soy Oil
Safflower Oil   Sesame Oil
Sunflower Oil

MILDLY STARCHY VEGETABLES

Artichokes
Beets
Carrots
Cauliflower
Corn
Peas

Excellent — Good — Poor — Fair

Fruits are best when eaten separate from other foods on an empty stomach. It is best to eat melons and sweet fruits separately. Fruit makes an awesome breakfast and an energetic start to the day.

ACID FRUITS		SUB ACID FRUITS		SWEET FRUITS		MELONS
Lemon	Lime	Apples	Pears	Bananas	Raisins	Cantaloupe
Orange	Tangerines	Cherries	Nectarines	Grapes	Prunes	Honey dew
Raspberries	Pomegranate	Tart Grapes	Mangoes	Dried fruits	Figs	Watermelon
Pineapple	Grapefruit	Huckleberries	Sweet Plums	Dates		Casaba
Blackberries	Strawberries	Kiwi	Apricots			Musk
Kumquat	Sour Plums	Papaya	Fresh Figs			Persian
Sour apples		Peach				Crenshaw

*Chapter Ten ...

Science of Nutrition*

****

Nutrition builds on two areas of Science - the Life Sciences covered in Biochemistry and the science of Physiology which tells us how Nutrition correlates to our physical health and body function.

The Behavioral Sciences help us understand how Nutrition is interwoven with our Psychosocial needs. Both aspects are at work in our lives.

We Human Organisms are highly complex groupings of Chemical Compounds that are constantly at work in an array of reactions that sustain Life. Nutrients participate in and help control these Chemical reactions. Various Physiologic systems integrate the activities of millions of functioning Cells, uniting them into a functioning whole. This highly sensitive internal control is called **Homeostasis**.

We also have social and emotional qualities rooted in our earliest awareness. Eating patterns and attitudes toward food develop over a lifetime based on the influences of our primary family and friends, ethnic or cultural group, community, nation, and world. How we perceive food, what we choose to eat, why we eat what we do, and the ways in which we eat are all integral to human nutrition.

Nutrition means *to nourish* and encompasses the food people eat and how it enriches their lives physically, socially, and personally. From the moment of conception until death, an appropriate supply of food supports optimal growth and maturation and mental and physical well-being.

Good nutrition promotes health and reduces the risk of adverse conditions ranging from low birth weight to obesity to cardiovascular disease.

Food supplies the energy to carry out body functions, such as inhaling and exhaling, maintaining body temperature, and engaging in physical activity.

Food also nourishes our Human Spirit. We all have our particular "soul foods," or comfort foods that connect us to our family and provide a sense of psychological and emotional well-being.

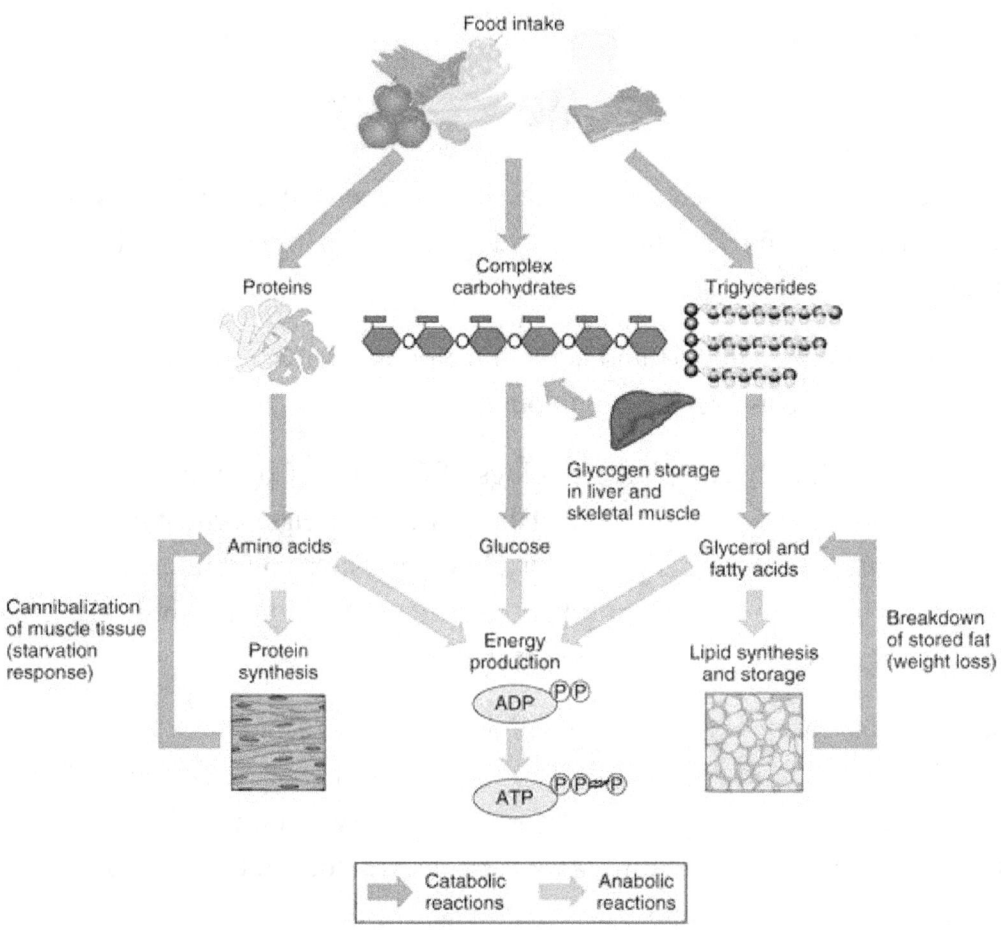

To study Nutrition, we need to define the terms that describe this body of knowledge and the health professionals who work within it. *Nutrition* refers to the food people eat and how it nourishes their bodies, whereas **Nutrition Science** defines the Nutrient requirements for Body Maintenance, Growth, Activity, and Reproduction.

Dietetics is the health profession with primary responsibility for the practical application of nutrition science throughout the life cycle in health and disease.

The **Registered Dietitian (RD) or Registered Dietitian Nutritionist (RDN)** is the nutrition expert on the health care team, and in collaboration with the physician and nurse, carries the major responsibility for a patient's nutritional care.

Public Health Nutritionists focus on disease prevention and oversee programs that serve high-risk groups in the community such as pregnant teens or older adults, assessing needs, and applying interventions. RDs cooperate with school nurses to teach weight-management classes for children and parents, assist day care providers in planning menus and snacks, or help clients at fitness centers improve their body composition or athletic performance.

Functions of Food and Nutrients

Food serves as the vehicle for bringing **Nutrients** into the body; however, the specific chemical compounds and elements in food—the nutrients—are the substances the body needs. No one particular food or food combination is required to ensure health. The human race has survived for centuries on a wide variety of foods, depending on what was available and what the culture designated as appropriate.

Approximately 50 Nutrients are known to be essential to human life and health, although countless other Elements and Molecules are being studied and may be found to be essential. The identification of an **Essential Nutrient** is especially important when developing liquid formulas for feeding critically ill patients.

Essential Nutrients include the **Macronutrients (Carbohydrates, Fats,** and **Proteins),** the **Micronutrients (Vitamins** and **Minerals),** and **Water**.

The Macronutrients supply Energy and build Tissue, whereas the Micronutrients, needed in much smaller amounts, form specialized structures and regulate body processes. Water is the additional and often-forgotten nutrient that sustains all life systems.

The sum of all the Chemical reactions occurring in the body that use nutrients is referred to as **Metabolism**. The first section of this text defines the Essential Nutrients; later chapters describe how they participate in growth, maturation, aging, and diet interventions in health and disease.

<u>*Nutrients have three general functions, as follows*</u>:

1. To provide energy

2. To build and repair body tissues and structures

3. To regulate the metabolic processes that maintain homeostasis.

Energy

All three of the Macronutrients—Carbohydrate, Fat, and Protein—can be used for energy, although Carbohydrates are your bodies preferred energy sources.

Carbohydrates

Dietary Carbs—Starch and Sugars—are the Primary Sources of fuel for Heat and Energy. Glucose, the break-down product of dietary Carbs, is the Energy currency of our bodies. *Glycogen* is the storage form of Carbohydrate available for quick energy when Glucose is needed.

Each gram of Carbohydrate when metabolized in the body yields 4 Kcals, known as its **Fuel Factor**.

In a well-balanced diet for a healthy person, 45% to 65% of total kcals come from carbs. The *majority* of these kcals should be obtained from Complex Carbohydrates (Starch), with a *smaller* amount from Simple Carbohydrates (Sugars). Another form of complex Carbohydrate, known as *Fiber,* does not yield Energy but has other important body functions.

Although the general public uses the word *calorie* to refer to the energy value of food, nutritionists use the technical term *kilocalorie*.

Fats

Dietary Fats from either animal or plant sources provide an alternate or storage form of energy. Fat is a more concentrated fuel than Carbs, with a fuel factor of 9, yielding 9 kcal/g. Most nutrition experts recommend that Fats supply no more than 20% to 35% of total kcals.

Fats contain the Essential Fatty Acids required for life and health. Saturated Fats are a *less* healthy form of Fat; therefore, the *majority* of our Fat intake should be Unsaturated.

Proteins

The primary function of Protein is Tissue Building, although it can be used for Energy if needed. The body draws on dietary or tissue Protein for Energy when the fuel supply from Carbohydrates and Fats is not sufficient to meet body needs.

Protein yields 4 kcal/g, making its fuel factor 4.

Protein can provide 10% to 35% of total kcals in a well-balanced diet for healthy people. Proteins also form vital substances such as enzymes and hormones that regulate body systems.

Minerals

Minerals help build tissues with very specific functions. The major Minerals—Calcium and Phosphorus—give strength to our Bones and Teeth.

The trace element Iron is a component of our Hemoglobin and binds Oxygen for transport to our Cells and Carbon Dioxide for return to our Lungs to be Exhaled out.

Minerals serve as cofactors in controlling our Cell Metabolism. One example is Iron, which controls the Enzyme actions in our Cell Mitochondria that produce and store high-energy compounds.

Vitamins

Vitamins are classified as Complex Molecules that are needed in very ***minute*** amounts but are essential in certain Tissues. There are many Vitamins that are components of our Cell Enzyme systems. They govern reactions that produce energy and **synthesize** important Molecules. For example, the element Thiamin controls the release of energy for our Cell work and Vitamin B_{12} is needed for the synthesis and maturation of our Red Blood Cells.

Vitamin C produces the Intercellular ground substance that cements our Tissues together and prevents Tissue bleeding.

Vitamin A is in the Rods and Cones of our Eyes and is needed for our Vision in dim light.

Metabolic Regulation

There are specific Vitamins and Minerals that are necessary for Enzyme activities responsible for a host of chemical reactions. Water provides the appropriate environment for these reactions to occur.

Water

Water forms our Blood, Lymph, and Intercellular fluids that transport our Nutrients to our Cells and removes waste. Water also functions as a Regulatory Agent, providing the fluid environment in which all metabolic reactions take place.

An important principle in nutrition is *Nutrient Interaction*. It has the following two parts:

1. Individual nutrients participate in many different metabolic functions; for some functions a nutrient has a primary role, and for others, it has a supporting role.

2. No nutrient ever works alone.

Intimate and ongoing metabolic relationships exist among all the nutrients and their **Metabolites**. Although we look at each nutrient individually to simplify our study, they do not exist that way in the body.

Nutrients are always working together within an integrated whole, providing Energy, Building and Rebuilding Tissue, and Regulating Metabolic activities.

This synergy and interaction among nutrients is important in carrying out body functions and is sometimes overlooked when we examine the effects of one nutrient at a time.

Nutritional Status

The Nutritional Health of an individual is known as his or her *Nutritional Status* and describes how well nutrient needs are being met. Nutritional Status is influenced by living situation, social and economic factors, available food, food choices, and state of health as well as the access to Quality foods.

Growing our own food is very inexpensive and eliminates several of the key factors listed above that can have a negative impact on our ability to eat High Energy foods.

Nutritional Status differs from *Dietary Status*. Evaluating Nutritional Status requires a combination of dietary, biochemical, Anthropometric, and clinical measurements, whereas dietary status focuses only on what foods are being consumed and their nutrient content.

 It is important to know not only what an individual is eating, but also whether the body is absorbing and making use of those nutrients.

This helps us distinguish between a *Primary Nutrient Deficiency* and a *Secondary Nutrient Deficiency*. A primary nutrient deficiency is caused by insufficient dietary intake of a particular nutrient or nutrients.

A secondary nutrient deficiency is the result of poor absorption or metabolism of a nutrient caused by an interfering substance, a disease or condition, or an elevated requirement.

Optimal Nutrition

Individuals with Optimal Nutritional status have *neither* a deficiency nor an excess of nutrients. Nutrient stores are at the upper end of the normal range. Evidence of Optimal Nutrition includes appropriate weight for height and good muscle development and tone. The skin is smooth, and the eyes are clear and bright. Appetite, digestion, and elimination are normal.

Well-nourished persons are more likely to be alert, both mentally and physically. They are not only meeting their day-to-day needs, but also maintaining appropriate nutrient stores to resist disease and support body function in times of stress.

Undernutrition

Undernutrition takes various forms ranging from marginal nutritional status to the emaciated famine victim. Persons with *Marginal Nutritional status* are meeting their minimum day-to-day nutritional needs but lack the nutrient stores to cope with any added physiologic or metabolic demand arising from injury or illness, pregnancy, or growth spurt. Marginal nutritional status results from poor eating habits, stressful environments, or insufficient resources to obtain appropriate types or amounts of food.

Current U.S. food trends add to the risk of marginal nutritional status or undernutrition among all age groups. Money spent for food away from home has increased, while money spent for food eaten at home has decreased by almost half.

Meals away from home, especially those obtained at fast-food restaurants, tend to be high in fat, sodium, and added sugar, but limited in calcium, fiber, whole grains, fruits, and green, yellow, and orange vegetables. Foods contributing the most kcals to the diets of persons ages 2 and over are grain-based desserts (cookies, cake, doughnuts, and granola bars), followed by yeast breads, chicken and chicken-mixed dishes, sugar-sweetened soft drinks, and pizza.

Sugar-sweetened soft drinks and fruit drinks supply almost half of the added sugar in the U.S. diet, and sugar intakes are times higher than recommended in the 2010 *Dietary Guidelines for Americans*. **Added sugar contributes 316 kcal per day to the average diet and is believed by some nutrition experts to be a major contributor to the obesity epidemic and rise in type 2 diabetes.**

Despite an abundance of kcalories, most Americans are deficient in Calcium, Vitamin D, Fiber, and Potassium.

Public health nutritionists describe the American diet as energy rich but nutrient poor. Although persons with less-than-optimal intakes of Micronutrients may not suffer from overt malnutrition, they are at greater risk of physical illness than those who are well nourished. The body can adapt to Marginal Nutrient intake but any added Physiologic Stress that calls on Nutrient stores will result in **overt malnutrition**.

Overnutrition

Overnutrition takes various forms. Excessive energy intake coupled with low physical activity leads to unwanted weight gain and elevated health risks for conditions such as metabolic syndrome.

Overnutrition also occurs with *excessive* intakes of Micronutrients from overuse of dietary supplements.

Inappropriate amounts of particular Vitamins or Minerals damage tissues and interfere with the absorption and metabolism of other essential nutrients.

Herbal preparations, growing in popularity, carry the potential for harmful interactions with nutrients or medications.

Nutrient Density

A major factor in our nutritional health is the *Nutrient Density* of the diet. This term refers to the relative Nutrient content of a food in relation to its Energy content.

A **Nutrient-Dense** food contributes Vitamins, Minerals, Essential Fatty Acids, and/or Protein to the diet in addition to their specific kcals.

A food that is not nutrient dense adds kcals but lacks other vital Life Nutrients. A hamburger made from lean ground beef supplies protein and many vitamins and minerals, although it adds some fat.

Fruits and vegetables high in Vitamins and Minerals and low in kcals are Nutrient Dense. Those that we grow and harvest ourselves manifest the Highest amount of Life Energy.

In contrast, a doughnut high in kcalories adds primarily TOXIC Sugar and Fat, and sugar-sweetened soft drinks add only TOXIC kcals. These foods we consider to be "**empty calories**" as they contribute no Essential Nutrients. *Many Americans who are overweight or obese exhibit undernutrition because the foods they consume are not nutrient dense.*

Nutrition Standards

Dietary Reference Intakes

Most countries have standards for nutrient intakes of healthy people according to age and sex. Health professionals use these standards in making decisions about the nutritional health of individuals and groups. In the U.S., these nutrient and energy standards are called the Dietary Reference Intakes (DRIs), and include several categories of recommendations.

Each category within the DRIs has a different purpose and use for the Health and Nutritional Professional. Each of these terms is described below:

• *Dietary Reference Intakes (DRIs):* The U.S. framework of nutrient standards that provide reference values for use in planning and evaluating diets for healthy people. The DRIs include the recommended dietary allowance, the adequate intake, the tolerable upper intake level, and the estimated average requirement.

• ***Recommended Dietary Allowance (RDA):*** The average daily intake of a nutrient that will meet the requirement of 97% to 98% (or two standard deviations of the mean) of healthy people of a given age and sex.

The RDAs were established and are reviewed periodically by an expert panel of nutrition scientists; they are amended as needed based on new research findings. RDAs have been set for Carbs, Protein, Essential Fatty acids, and most vitamins and minerals. When planning diets the RDA serves as an intake goal.

• ***Adequate Intake (AI):*** A suggested daily intake of a nutrient to meet body needs and support health. The AI is used when there is not sufficient research available to develop an RDA but the nutrient appears to have a strong health benefit. The AI serves as a guide for intake when planning diets.

• *Tolerable Upper Intake Level (UL):* The highest amount of a nutrient that can be consumed safely with no risk of toxicity or adverse effects. The UL is used to evaluate the nutrient content of dietary supplements or review total nutrient intake from food and supplements. Intakes exceeding the UL usually result from concentrated supplements, not food.

• ***Estimated Average Requirement (EAR):*** The average daily intake of a nutrient that will meet the requirement of 50% of healthy people of a given age and sex. The EAR is used to plan and evaluate the nutrient intakes of groups rather than individuals.

• *Acceptable Macronutrient Distribution Range (AMDR):* The AMDR guides the division of kcals among Carbs, Fats, and Protein in ranges supportive of building optimal health; Carbs should provide 45% to 65% of total kcals, Fat should provide 20% to 35% of total kcals, and Protein should provide 10% to 35% of total kcals.

The DRIs for vitamins, minerals, and macronutrients can be found on the inside front cover and first page of this text. Note there are two age categories for persons over age 50, directing our attention to the changes in nutrient requirements as we age.

The first set of DRIs, replacing earlier RDAs, was released in 1997. These guidelines provided new standards for Calcium, Phosphorus, Magnesium, and Vitamin D and emphasized the role of these Nutrients in our Bone health. Since then, DRIs have been established for the B-complex Vitamins (1998); Anti-Oxidant Nutrients and Carotenoids (2000); Vitamins A and K and the trace Minerals (2001); energy, the energy-yielding Macronutrients, and Fiber (2002); and Electrolytes and Water (2004).

The DRIs for Calcium and Vitamin D were revised again in 2010, based on new evidence indicating increased needs for bone health.

The nutrient standards of Canada and Great Britain are similar to those of the U.S. Developing countries use standards set by the United Nations Food and Agriculture Organization (FAO).

1. Substitute lower calorie, nutrient-dense foods for refined grains and snack foods high in Solid Fat and Sugar (SoFAS). ***Move to a more plant-based diet by adding fruits, vegetables, whole grains, peas, and beans***. These foods, along with fat-free, low-fat, or reduced-fat dairy products, will raise intakes of Potassium, Calcium, Fiber, and Vitamin D, now inadequate in many American diets.

These finding support the need and importance of growing and harvesting our own Food. Each of the recommendations of a Plant-Based diet can be produced in our own Garden = Access to the Highest Quality of Life Energy = Increase our Success of Building our Supreme Health = Enjoying Abundant Life !!!!

2. The Minerals Sodium and Potassium are known to have opposite effects on our Blood Pressure, with Potassium blunting the blood-pressure-raising effect of sodium. The 2005 *DGA* recommended a sodium intake of no more than 2300 mg/day (the UL for sodium) for the general population, but ***noted that hypertensive individuals, African Americans, and middle-aged and older individuals would benefit from reducing their intakes to 1500 mg/day or less (the AI for sodium***). Because these groups now comprise a major proportion of U.S. adults, the Advisory Committee recommended a goal of 1500 mg/day of Sodium for the general population.

However, given the current high Sodium content of food in the marketplace and the taste perception of the general public, the decrease from 2300 mg to 1500 mg will need to occur gradually over time. ***Because Blood Pressure-related Atherosclerotic disease begins in childhood, both children and adults must lower their Sodium intake.***

Eating other-than-Human foods introduces TOXICITY into our Bodies which contributes to a significant decrease our Life Energy. This is happening with a simultaneous increase in our chances of being detrimentally affected and suffering from the associated health issues from eating these non-human foods or elements.

Whole Wheat Bread

Nutrition Facts	Amount/Serving	%DV*	Amount/Serving	%DV*
Serving Size 1 Slice (27g)	Total Fat 1g	2%	Total Carb. 12g	4%
Servings Per Container 17	Sat. Fat 0g	0%	Dietary Fiber 2g	8%
Calories 70	Trans Fat 0g	0%	Sugars 2g	
Calories from Fat 10	Cholesterol 0mg	0%	Protein 2g	
	Sodium 10mg	0%		

*Percent Daily Values (DV) are based on a 2,000-calorie diet. Your daily values may be higher or lower depending on your calorie needs.

	Calories:	2,000	2,500
Total Fat	Less than	65g	80g
Sat Fat	Less than	20g	25g
Cholesterol	Less than	300mg	300mg
Sodium	Less than	2,400mg	2,400mg
Total Carbohydrate		300g	375g
Dietary Fiber		25g	30g

Vitamin A 0% • Vitamin C 0% • Calcium 4% • Iron 4%
Thiamin 4% • Riboflavin 2% • Niacin 4%

INGREDIENTS: WHOLE WHEAT FLOUR, WATER, MOLASSES, WHEAT GLUTEN, SOYBEAN. CONTAINS 2% OR LESS OF THE FOLLOWING: YEAST, DOUGH CONDITIONERS (MONO DIGLYCERIDES, ETHOXYLATED MONO & GLYCERIDES, CALCIUM STEAROYL-2-LACTYLATE), YEAST NUTRIENTS (CALCIUM SULFATE, MONO- CALCIUM PHOSPHATE), CALCIUM PROPIONATE (A PRESERVATIVE).

The Nutrition Facts panel of a food label lists the number of grams of total carbohydrate and fiber and gives these amounts as a percentage of the Daily Value.

The Daily Value for total carbohydrate is 60% of the diet's energy content, or 300 g for a 2000-Calorie diet. The Daily Value for fiber in a 2000-Calorie diet is 25 g.

To identify products made mostly from *whole* grains, look for the word "whole" before the name of the grain. If this is the first ingredient listed, the product is made from mostly wheat, not whole wheat. Note that foods labeled with the words "multigrain", "stone-ground", "100% wheat," "cracked wheat," "seven-grain," or "bran" are not necessarily 100% whole-grain products and may not contain any whole grains.

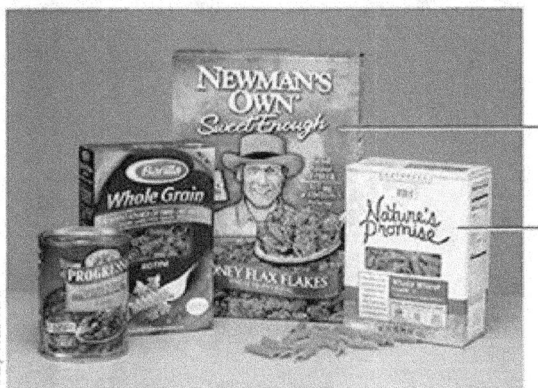

Foods labeled "high fiber" contain 20% or more of the Daily Value per serving.

Foods labeled "good source of fiber" contain between 10 and 19% of the Daily Value per serving.

Products labeled "reduced sugar" contain 25% less sugar than the regular, or reference, product.

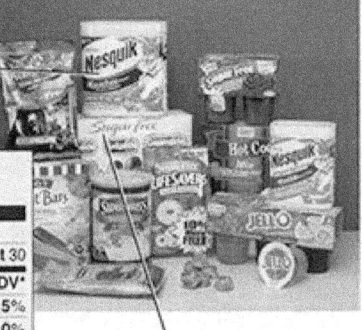

The ingredient list helps identify added sugars. Many products have more than one added sweetener. The closer the name of each sweetener appears to the beginning of the list, the more of it has been added.

INGREDIENTS: CULTURED PASTEURIZED GRADE A REDUCED FAT MILK, SUGAR, NONFAT MILK, HIGH FRUCTOSE CORN SYRUP, STRAWBERRY PUREE, MODIFIED CORN STARCH, KOSHER GELATIN, TRI-CALCIUM PHOSPHATE, NATURAL FLAVOR, COLORED WITH CARMINE, VITAMIN A ACETATE, VITAMIN D3.

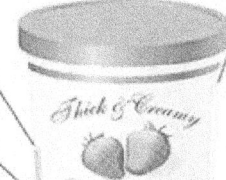

On the ingredient list, all these are added sugar: Brown sugar, corn sweetener, corn syrup, dextrose, fructose, fruit juice, glucose, high fructose corn syrup, honey, invert sugar, lactose, maltose, malt syrup, molasses, raw sugar, sucrose, and sugar syrup concentrates.

Nutrition Facts
Serving Size 1 Container

Amount Per Serving	
Calories 190	Calories from Fat 30

Amount/Serving	% DV*
Total Fat 3.5g	5%
Saturated Fat 2g	10%
Trans Fat 0g	
Cholesterol 15mg	4%
Sodium 100mg	4%
Potassium 310mg	9%
Total Carbohydrate 32g	11%
Dietary Fiber 0g	0%
Sugars 28g	
Protein 7g	14%

Vitamin A 15% • Calcium 30%

*Percent Daily Values (DV) are based on a 2,000 calorie diet.

Foods labeled "sugar free" contain less than 0.5 g of sugar per serving.

The number of grams of sugars listed includes the total amounts of mono- and disaccharides but does not distinguish between added sugar and the sugar that occurs naturally in the food. Proposed changes to the Nutrition Facts include putting grams of added sugars as a separate line below Sugars.

*Chapter Eleven....

How Safe Is Your Food Supply?*

****

Americans believe that much, if not all, of the food they purchase has been inspected for safety, and that the facilities in which their food is prepared and processed are certified to be sanitary and disease- and contaminate-free. Of course it is cost-prohibitive and impractical to inspect every single facility and every product every minute of every day, so sometimes food reaches us that is not safe. *And sometimes it reaches us completely uninspected by anyone.*

This is why it is of the upmost importance that we Grow Our Own FOOD!! Food is our source of Life Energy and we can only Grow and Develop as our food is Grown and Developed.

Organic food production

Organic food is produced using methods that minimize the use of synthetic pesticides and promote recycling of resources and conservation of Soil and Water to protect the environment. The USDA sets standards for substances that can be used in or are prohibited from use in organic food production.

Most conventional pesticides, fertilizers made with synthetic ingredients, sewage sludge, genetically modified ingredients, irradiation, antibiotics, and growth hormones are prohibited from use in organic food production.

Before a food can be labeled "***Organic***," the USDA must certify the farming and processing operations that produce and handle the food.

Organic Food- Food that is Produced, Processed, and Handled in accordance with the standards of the USDA National Organic Program.

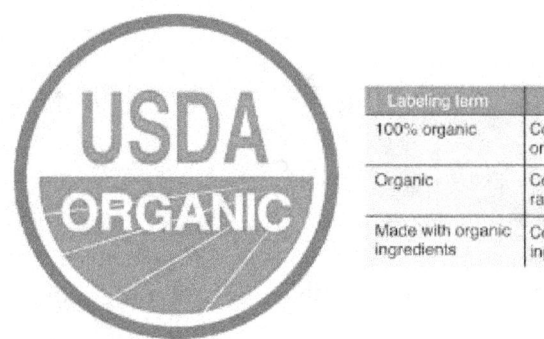

Labeling term	Meaning
100% organic	Contains 100% organically produced raw or processed ingredients.
Organic	Contains at least 95% organically produced raw or processed ingredients.
Made with organic ingredients	Contains at least 70% organically produced ingredients.

The term ORGANIC is an Advertising and Marketing word, used to increase the Profit of food manufactureres….NOT to ensure that we are buying/consuming Naturally occurring or Grown Food.

Labeling organic foods

Products that meet the definition of "*100% Organic*" or "*Organic*" may display the USDA "*Organic*" seal shown here.

Organic farming techniques reduce farm workers' exposure to pesticides and decrease the quantity of pesticides introduced into the food supply and the environment.

Organic foods, however, are not completely free of synthetic pesticides and other agricultural chemicals not approved for organic use because irrigation water, rain, and a variety of other sources can introduce trace amounts into organically grown foods.

The threshold for pesticide residues in organic foods is set at 5% of the EPA's pesticide-residue tolerance.

Choosing organic food will reduce pesticide exposure, but it will not make your food risk free.

The ONLY way to be 100% sure that we are eating Pesticide free and Organically Grown and Harvested food is to GROW OUR OWN FOOD!

Bio-Technology

Biotechnology alters the characteristics of organisms by making selective changes in their DNA. The concept is not new. For centuries, farmers have selected seeds from plants with the most desirable characteristics to plant for the next year's crop, bred the animals that grew fastest or produced the most milk to improve the productivity of the next generation of animals, and crossbred plant varieties to combine the desired traits of each. However, these traditional methods may require many generations to produce the desired results. Biotechnology uses **Genetic Engineering** or **Genetic Modification (GM)** to select genes for specific traits. Genetic Engineering has significantly sped up the process of modifying the traits of organisms.

Like all other new technologies, however, it may introduce new risks because WE ARE WHAT WE EAT. Eating Genetically Modified food items releases Genetically Modified ENRGY = TOXIC Energy!

Bio-Technology

Bio-technology- Is the process of manipulating Life forms through Genetic Engineering in order to produce, manufacture and provide desirable products for human use.

Genetic Engineering or **Genetic Modification (GM)** is a set of techniques used to manipulate the DNA of an Organism for the purpose of changing the Characteristics of that specific organism for creating a new Element.

You Are What You EAT!!!!!

For EVERY Action There Is An OPPOSITE and EQUAL Re-Action….Consuming a Genetically Engineered/Modified food item causes an Opposite and Equal Genetic Engineering IN YOU !!!!

Could this be WHY there is a Health Crisis of a RISE in Dis-eases, illnesses and pre-mature Death?

WHO is Growing the Food YOU EAT?

HOW are they Growing the Food YOU EAT?

How Biotechnology Works

Genetically Modified Organism (GMO) are made through Genetic Engineering. To modify a plant such as corn, a piece of DNA containing the Gene for a desired characteristic is taken from Plant, Animal, or Bacterial Cells and Transferred to corn plant Cells.

This DNA is now classified and referred to as **Recombinant DNA** because the new DNA is a combination of the DNA from two different Organisms.

The modified corn cells are then allowed to *divide* into more and more Cells and eventually differentiate into the various types of Cells that make up a whole corn plant. *The new plant is a now considered to be scientifically classified as a Transgenic Organism.*

Each Cell in the new plant contains the Transferred Gene for the *desired trait*. This technique is used to introduce characteristics such as disease and drought resistance into plants.

Genetic Engineering is more difficult in animals because animal cells do not take up genes as easily as plant cells do, and making copies of these cells (clones) is also more difficult. *However, these techniques have been used to produce cows that yield more milk, cattle and pigs that have more meat on them, and sheep that grow more wool.*

Recombinant DNA - DNA that has been formed by joining DNA from different sources.

Transgenic - An organism with a Gene or group of Genes *intentionally* transferred from *another* Species or Breed.

HOW does these Genetically Modified Organisms EFFECT Humans when they EAT them?

Does this make YOU other than YOU God Created SELF?

Can this be the root cause to Human dis-ease, birth defects and pre-mature death?

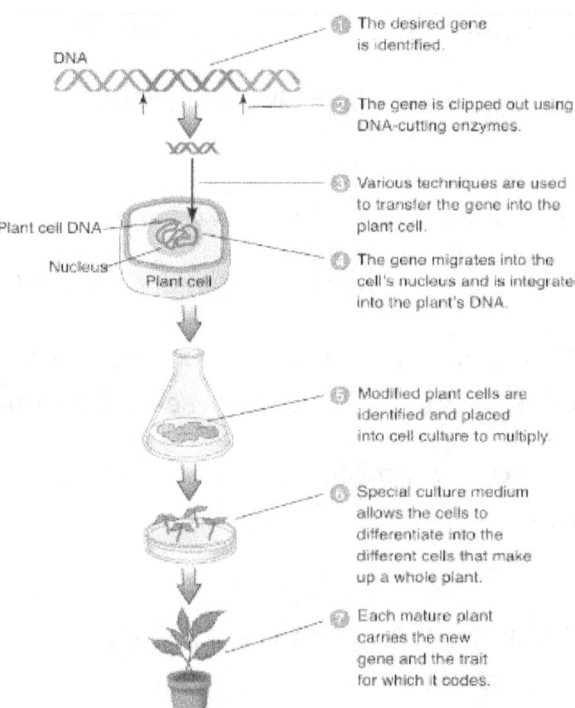

Biotechnology is also used in *Food Processing*. For example, many foods are produced with the help of man-made Enzymes. Rennet is an Enzyme used in *cheese production*; there are Enzymes used in the production of *High-Fructose Corn Syrup*; and the Enzyme Lactase is used to reduce the Natural Lactose content of milk, ___are now all produced by GM microbes___.

All of these food-like products are TOXIC and produce high levels of Toxicity in the eater.

Biotechnology is advertised as presenting great potential for addressing the problem of world hunger and malnutrition. *Although world hunger is rooted in political, economic, and cultural issues that cannot be resolved by agricultural technology alone*.

So instead of promoting the Natural idea of everyone Growing their Own Food, the Food Industry continues to develop un-natural GM crops that are advertised to target some of the major nutritional deficiencies worldwide are being developed.

Growing our own food almost immediately SOLVES the world hunger and malnutrition problem.

What better access to Natural food than right in your own yard?

How can there be a hunger issue with everyone having their own garden?

To address the advertised Protein deficiency, varieties of corn, soybeans, and sweet potatoes with enhanced levels of essential amino acids are being developed.

This is done DESPITE the fact Soybeans and Sweet Potatoes are NOT Human Food and are considerable TOXIC when consumed by us!

To address the advertised Vitamin A deficiency, Genes that are coded for the production of Enzymes needed for the synthesis of the Vitamin A precursor β-Carotene have been manufactured and un-naturally inserted into Rice.

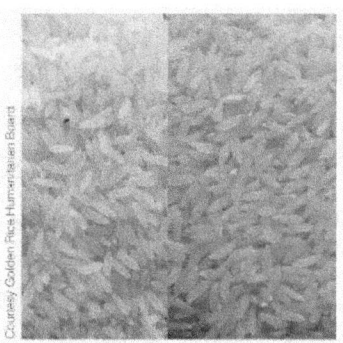

c. Half the world's population depends on rice as a dietary staple, but rice is a poor source of vitamin A. Genetically modified rice, called Golden Rice (seen here compared with white rice) for the color imparted by the β-carotene pigment, has the potential to significantly increase vitamin A intake (discussed further in Chapter 14 Debate). One variety contains enough provitamin A in 1 cup of cooked rice to meet the needs of a child.[48]

Vitamin A is a Naturally occurring by-product of the Life Energy from the Sun and is Naturally present in a variety of Fruits and Veggies that can be easily Grown and Harvested in our own Gardens.

SO WHY GENETICALLY ENGINEER AND MODIFY A NATURALLY OCCURING ELEMENT?

To address multiple advertised Nutrient deficiencies, the *BioCassava Plus program* has used the science of bio-technology to un-naturally develop Cassava with increased levels of Genetically Engineered and Modified Zinc, Iron, Protein, and Vitamin. All of which are MICRO-Nutrients, and too many of these elements can easily create a TOXIC environment in the Eater.

Risks and Regulation of Biotechnology

The rapid advancement of biotechnology during the past decade has created the potential for health problems and environmental damage. Regulations are in place to control the use of Genetic Engineering and GMOs.

Despite these precautions, many consumers and scientists believe that the impact of this booming technology has not yet become apparent. They urge that this technology be used with caution to avoid health or environmental impacts that outweigh the benefits.

Consumer concerns

Consumer safety concerns related to GM foods include the possibility that the nutrient content of a food may have been negatively affected or that an allergen or a toxin may have inadvertently been introduced into a food that was previously safe.

For example, if DNA from fish or nuts—foods that commonly cause allergic reactions—were introduced into soybeans or corn, these foods would then be dangerous to individuals allergic to fish or nuts.

Environmental concerns

An environmental concern about GM crops is that they will be used to the exclusion of other varieties, thereby reducing biodiversity. The ability of populations of organisms to adapt to new conditions, diseases, or other hazards depends on the presence of many different species and varieties that provide a diversity of genes.

If farmers plant only GM insect-resistant, high-yielding crops, other species and varieties may eventually become extinct, and the genes for the traits they possess may be lost forever.

Another environmental issue is the possibility that GM crops will create "superweeds."

This might occur, for example, if a Trait such as increased rate of growth introduced into a domesticated plant species were passed on to a related wild species. This could produce a fast-growing weed, or superweed, that would compete with the domesticated species.

There is also concern that crops that have been engineered to produce pesticides will promote the evolution of pesticide-resistant insects. An illustration is the case of insects that feed on plants modified to produce the Bt Toxin. As more and more of the insects' food supply consists of plants that produce this pesticide, only insects that carry genes that make them resistant to Bt Toxin survive and reproduce. This increases the number of

Bt-resistant insects and therefore reduces the effectiveness of Bt Toxin as a method of pest control.

Although an important concern when growing GM crops, pesticide-resistant insects may also evolve when pesticides are sprayed on crops.

Regulation of GM food products

The most common GM crops are soybeans, corn, cotton, and rapeseed (or canola). Therefore, foods produced in the United States that contain corn or high-fructose corn syrup, such as many breakfast cereals, snack foods, and soft drinks; foods made with soybeans; and foods made with cottonseed and canola oils are likely to contain GM ingredients.

This makes a majority of the American food supply non-human food = TOXIC when consumed by Humans!

Because of CLEVER advertising and specially created catch-phrases, we don't easily recognize these foods as Genetically Modified because they appear no different from other foods, and food manufacturers are **NOT** required to provide special labeling **unless** the food is known to pose a potential risk.

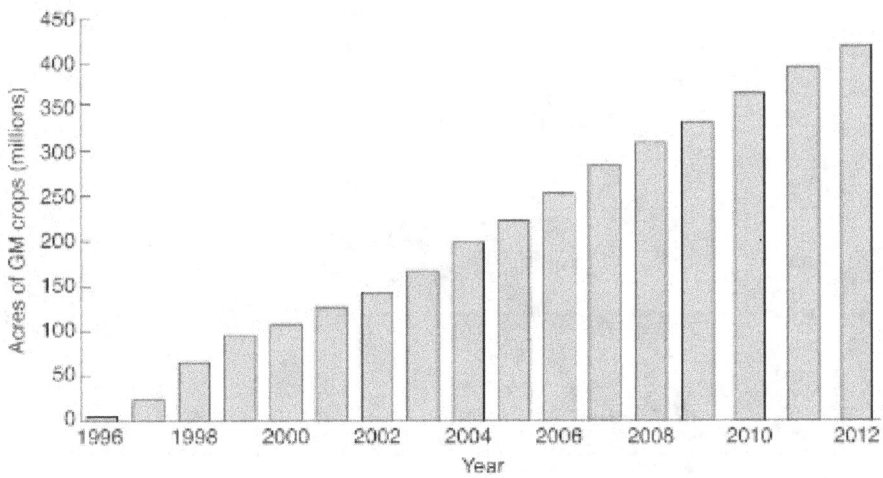

Growth of GM crops

Despite concerns about the impact of GM crops, the number of acres planted with them worldwide has risen steadily.

Food Irradiation

Food Irradiation, also called cold Pasteurization, is used in more than 40 countries to treat everything from frog legs to rice.

Irradiation exposes food to excessively high and un-natural doses of X-rays, Gamma Radiation, or High-Energy Electrons in order to kill microbes and insects and in-activate Natural Enzymes that cause Natural Germination and Ripening of fruits and veggies.

Because irradiation produces compounds that are not present in the original foods, it is treated as a food additive, and the level of radiation that may be used is regulated.

Irradiation- A process that exposes foods to Radiation in order to kill contaminating organisms and retard the ripening and spoilage of fruits and vegetables.

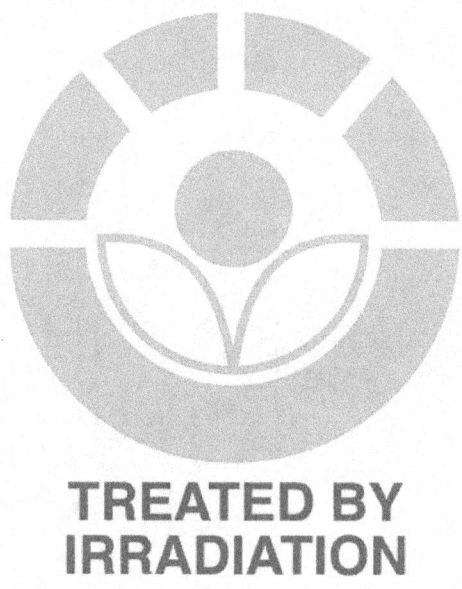

TREATED BY
IRRADIATION

Irradiated foods must be labeled with the **_Radura_** symbol shown above and the statement "**_treated with radiation_**" or "**_treated by irradiation_**."

This symbol is not required on the labels of foods that contain Irradiated spices or other Irradiated ingredients.

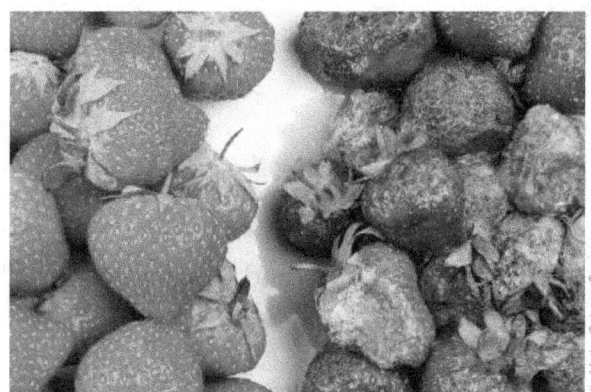

After 2 weeks in cold storage, the strawberries on the left, which were treated by **Irradiation**, remain free of mold, whereas the untreated strawberries on the right, which were picked at the same time, are covered with mold.

Food Packaging

Packaging plays an important role in food preservation; it keeps molds and bacteria out, keeps moisture in, and protects food from physical damage. An open package of refrigerated cheddar cheese will be moldy in a few days, but an unopened package will stay fresh for weeks.

Food packaging is continually being improved. In the past two decades, for instance, consumer demand for fresh and easy-to-prepare foods has led manufacturers to offer partially cooked pasta, vegetables, seafood, fresh and cured meats, and dry products such as whole-bean and ground coffee in packaging that, if unopened, will keep perishable food fresh much longer than will conventional packaging.

Vacuum packaging and **Modified Atmosphere Packaging (MAP)** use plastics or other packaging materials that are impermeable to oxygen. In vacuum packaging, the air inside *Page / 157* the package is removed prior to sealing in order to eliminate the oxygen.

In Modified Atmosphere Packaging, *the air is flushed out and replaced with another Gas, such as Carbon Dioxide, Sodium Dioxide or Nitrogen*.

Both Carbon Dioxide and Sodium Dioxide are scientifically classified as Poison = TOXIC when eaten!

Carbon Dioxide is Human WASTE Product!

In both of these types of packaging, the low Oxygen level prevents the growth of Aerobic bacteria, slows the ripening of fruits and vegetables, and slows down Oxidation reactions, which cause discoloration in fruits and vegetables and rancidity in fats.

Modified Atmosphere Packaging (MAP)- A preservation technique used to prolong the shelf life of processed or fresh food by changing the gases surrounding the food in the package.

Packaging can protect food from spoilage, but even the best packaging can introduce risk if it becomes part of the food. A variety of substances found in paper and plastic containers and packaging, and even dishes, can leach into food.

Substances that are known to contaminate food are regulated by the EPA and the FDA. However, these regulations apply only to the *intended* use of the product.

When a product is used improperly, substances from its packaging can migrate into food. For instance, some plastics migrate into food when heated in a microwave oven. Thus, only containers designed for microwave cooking should be used for microwaving food.

This science underscores the need to grow our own food so that we can have direcy access to Fresh Fruits and Veggies – Life Elements, WITHOUT the TOXIC packaging from commercial foods.

Page | 158

Bisphenol A from plastics

Bisphenol A (BPA) is a chemical in plastic that's used in hard, transparent water bottles, baby bottles, and food containers as well as the coating *inside* canned food items.

Some but not all plastic containers marked with recycle codes 3 or 7 are made with BPA.

There is some concern that BPA could adversely affect development in fetuses, infants, and children. The FDA supports efforts to eliminate the use of BPA in baby bottles and infant feeding cups and to replace BPA or minimize BPA levels in food can linings.

Aseptic processing

The juice boxes that fit so conveniently into school lunch bags are produced by Aseptic processing. This technique heats foods to temperatures that result in Sterilization. The sterilized foods are then placed in sterilized packages, using sterilized packaging equipment. If the package remains unopened, juice and other aseptically packaged foods can remain free of microbial growth at room temperature for years.

Preservation techniques that rely on temperature benefit consumers by providing appealing, safe foods, but these foods are not risk free, particularly if they are handled incorrectly.

If foods are not heated long enough or to a high enough temperature, or if they are not kept cold enough, they could pose a risk of food-borne illness. In addition, some types of cooking can generate hazardous chemicals.

Dangers of Eating Animal Meat

Carcinogenic Chemicals produced during the cooking of meats include Polycyclic Aromatic Hydrocarbons (PAHs) and Hetero-Cyclic Amines (HCAs).

PAHs are formed when fat drips on a grill and burns. They rise with the smoke and are deposited on the surface of the food.

PAH formation can be minimized by selecting lower-fat meat and using a layer of aluminum foil to prevent fat from dripping on the coals.

HCAs are produced by the burning of amino acids and other substances in meats and are formed during any type of high-temperature cooking.

HCA formation can be reduced by precooking meat, marinating meat before cooking, cooking at lower temperatures, and reducing cooking time by using smaller pieces of meat and avoiding overcooking.

The cooking temperatures recommended by the FDA are designed to prevent microbial food-borne illness and minimize the production of PAHs and HCAs.

Because PAHs and HCAs are considered accidental contaminants, their amounts in food are not regulated by the FDA.

This science supports that fact that Humans ARE HERBIVORES….the very process of cooking or even preparing animal meats turns their Energy TOXIC to the Human consumer!

Another contaminant formed during food preparation is **Acrylamide**. It is formed as a result of chemical reactions that occur during high-temperature baking or frying, particularly in carbohydrate-rich foods.

The highest levels of acrylamide are found in French fries and snack chips.

Smaller amounts are found in coffee and in foods made from grains, such as breakfast cereal and cookies.

High doses can cause cancer and reproductive problems in experimental animals and act as neurotoxins in humans.

Methods for reducing the amounts and potential Toxicity of Acrylamide in foods are being investigated.

Regulating Food Additives

Food additives are advertised to improve food quality and help protect us from disease, ***BUT if the wrong additive is used or the wrong amount is added, it could do more harm than good***.

A manufacturer that wants to use a new food additive must submit to the FDA a petition that describes the chemical composition of the additive, how it is manufactured, and how it is detected in food. The manufacturer must prove that the additive will be effective for its intended purpose at the proposed levels, that it is safe for its intended use, and that its use is necessary.

Additives may not be used to disguise inferior products or deceive consumers. They cannot be used if they significantly destroy nutrients or if the same effect can be achieved through sound manufacturing processes.

More than 600 chemicals defined as food additives were already in common use when legislation regulating food additives was passed. To accommodate substances that the FDA or the USDA had already determined to be safe, they were designated as **Prior-Sanctioned Substance** and are ***exempt*** from regulation.

The Nitrates and Nitrites used to retard the growth of *Clostridium Botulinum* in cured meats are Prior-Sanctioned Substances, for instance. ***However, their use has been controversial because they form carcinogenic nitrosamine in the digestive tract***. They are still allowed in foods, however, because they prevent botulism, and there is little evidence that they pose a serious risk in the amounts consumed in the human diet.

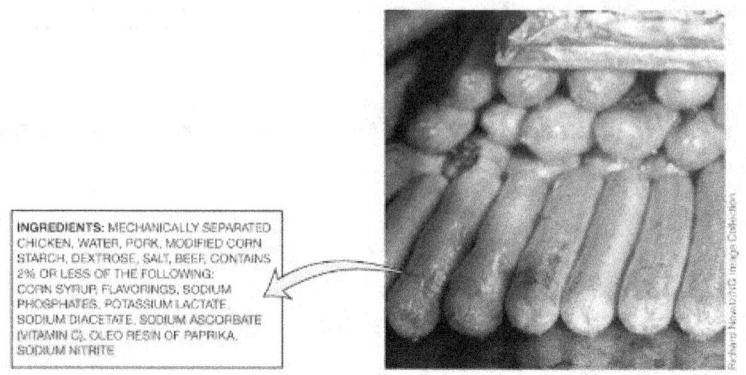

INGREDIENTS: MECHANICALLY SEPARATED CHICKEN, WATER, PORK, MODIFIED CORN STARCH, DEXTROSE, SALT, BEEF, CONTAINS 2% OR LESS OF THE FOLLOWING: CORN SYRUP, FLAVORINGS, SODIUM PHOSPHATES, POTASSIUM LACTATE, SODIUM DIACETATE, SODIUM ASCORBATE (VITAMIN C), OLEO RESIN OF PAPRIKA, SODIUM NITRITE

Understanding the science of these un-natural Substances and their wide-spread use in almost EVERY food-like product sold commercially allows us to make better Nutritional choices.

The Energy that is released from these synthetic elements is TOXIC to Human consumers.

Reducing Nitrosamine Risk

To minimize the risk posed by nitrosamines without increasing the risk of bacterial food-borne illness, the FDA limits the amount of Nitrate and Nitrite that can be added to food and requires the addition of antioxidants such as Vitamin C, which reduce Nitrosamine formation, to foods that contain these additives.

Consumers can reduce Nitrosamine exposure by limiting their consumption of cured meat to 3 to 4 ounces per week and maintaining adequate intakes of the antioxidant vitamins C and E.

A second category that is not subject to food additive regulation consists of substances **Generally Recognized As Safe (GRAS)**, based either on their history of use in food before 1958 or on published scientific evidence. *However, just because a substance is on the GRAS or prior-sanctioned list doesn't mean that it is safe or that it will stay on these lists.* If new evidence suggests that a substance in either category is unsafe, the

FDA **_may take action_** (but not necessarily) to require that the substance be removed from food products.

Generally Recognized As Safe (GRAS) - A group of Chemical Additives that are considered safe, based on their longstanding presence in the food supply without harmful *Page | 162* effects.

Substances that are toxic at some level of consumption may be harmless at a lower level. To ensure that additives are safe, most of those that are allowed in foods can be added only at levels 100 times below the highest level that has been shown to have no harmful effects.

Identifying Food Additives

Food Additives are used to make food safer; maintain palatability and wholesomeness; improve color, flavor, or texture; aid in processing; and enhance nutritional value. Their use ensures the availability of wholesome, appetizing, and affordable foods that meet consumer demands throughout the year.

The FDA's database *Everything Added to Food in the United States* lists more than 3000 additives. Many of these, such as sugar and spices, are used in homes every day.

Other additives may sound like a chemical soup: calcium propionate in bread, disodium EDTA in kidney beans, and BHA in potato chips.

Understanding what these chemicals are used for can help make the ingredient list a source of information rather than a cause for concern.

Sensitivities to Additives

Some individuals are allergic or sensitive to certain food additives. For example, the Flavor Enhancer – Mono-Sodium Glutamate (MSG), commonly used in Chinese food, can cause adverse reactions known as *MSG Symptom Complex* or *Chinese Restaurant Syndrome* in sensitive individuals. Sulfites can cause symptoms ranging from stomachache and hives to severe asthma.

Sulfites are used as preservatives in baked goods, canned foods, condiments, and dried fruits. Sensitive individuals can identify foods that contain sulfites by checking food labels.

Understanding that this significantly TOXIC element is used in almost every form of commercial food should high-light the Importance of Growing our own FOOD!

The forms of Sulfites allowed in packaged foods include: Sulfur Dioxide, Sodium Sulfite, Sodium and Potassium Bisulfite, and Sodium and Potassium Metabisulfite.

Almost ALL Foods served in restaurants may also contain sulfites. For example, a potato dish served in a restaurant may be prepared using potatoes that were peeled and soaked in a Sulfite Solution *before* cooking.

Color Additives are also clinically known to also cause adverse reactions. For example, FD&C Yellow No. 5, also conspicuously listed as Tartrazine on Medicine Labels, may cause itching and hives in sensitive people. It is found in beverages, desserts, and processed vegetables.

Color additives are listed in the ingredient list along with other food additives. Colors in foods are classified as *certified* or *exempt*. Certified Colors are man-made and are required to meet strict specifications for purity and must be listed by name in the ingredient list.

Colors that are exempt from certification include Pigments from Natural Sources such as Dehydrated Beets and Carotenoids; these may be listed collectively in the ingredient list as "*artificial color.*"

Antibiotics & Hormones

Antibiotics and hormones are administered to animals to improve health, increase growth, or otherwise enhance food production. To attempt to prevent these potentially toxic to Human chemicals from being passed on to consumers, both the types of drugs used and when they can be administered are regulated, and animal tissues are monitored for drug residues.

Animals are treated with Antibiotics when they are sick, but for decades animals have also been given antibiotics to prevent disease and promote growth. *This treatment increases the amount of meat produced and reduces costs, but if it is used improperly, antibiotic residues can remain in the meat. In addition, the overuse of antibiotics in animals can contribute to the development of antibiotic-resistant strains of bacteria.*

When exposed to an antibiotic, bacteria that are resistant to it survive and produce offspring that are also resistant. If these antibiotic-resistant bacteria infect humans, the resulting illness cannot be treated with that antibiotic.

Humans ARE HERBIVORES and the afore-mentioned conditions manifest from eating other-than-Human foods…..which in-turn creates other-than-Human dis-eases and ther health conditions – like Tuberculosis!

In order to limit antibiotic use, in 2013, the FDA took steps that will make the use of Antibiotics for growth enhancement of healthy livestock illegal; antibiotics will still be available to treat sick animals, but only with a veterinary prescription. These are great intentions, but the unfortunate aspect is that violators aren't caught/penalized until AFTER their product seriously injures or kills the Human eater.

Hormones are used to increase weight gain in sheep and cattle and milk production in dairy cows. Some hormones, such as Estrogen and Testosterone, occur naturally. Generally, these are administered in slow-release form, and their levels are no higher in treated animals than in untreated animals. Before a synthetic hormone can be used, it must be demonstrated that hormone residues in meat from treated animals are within safe limits.

Again, the unfortunate aspect is that violators aren't pursued until AFTER an injury or death!

A Synthetic Hormone that has created public concern is genetically engineered **Bovine Somatotropin (bST)**. Cows naturally produce bST, which stimulates milk production. Genetically engineered bST is produced by un-naturally by manufacturing Bacteria and injecting it into the cows to further increase milk production.

Milk from cows that have been treated with genetically engineered bST is indistinguishable from other milk by sight and taste – but the Energy that is released from the Genetically Modified milk is TOXIC when consumed by Humans.

When people have issues with a milk-based product, this synthetic hormone – Bovine Somatotropin may be the root cause and NOT Lactose.

Industrial Contaminants

Industrial Chemicals that contaminate the environment ultimately find their way into the food supply. Especially given the scientific fact that NOTHING leaves the Earth. Fish accumulate substances from the water in which they live and feed. Shellfish accumulate contaminants because they feed by passing large volumes of water through their bodies. Pollutants in the water can also contaminate crops and move through the food chain into meat and milk.

One group of Carcinogenic Compounds that pollutes the environment is **Poly-Chlorinated Biphenyls (PCBs)**. Prior to the 1970s, these chemicals were used in the manufacture of electrical capacitors and transformers, plasticizers, waxes, and paper. PCBs in runoff from manufacturing plants contaminated water, particularly near the Great Lakes.

PCBs are no longer produced, but because they do not degrade, they are still in the environment and accumulate in fish caught in contaminated waters. PCBs are a particular problem for pregnant and lactating women because prenatal exposure to

PCBs and consumption of contaminated breast milk can damage the fetal and infant nervous system and cause learning deficits.

Pregnant and breastfeeding women should check with their local health department for recommendations regarding fish consumption.

Humans ARE HERBIVORES !!

Other contaminants from the manufacturing process include elements such as Chlordane (used to control termites); Radioactive Substances such as Strontium-90; and toxic metals such as Cadmium, Lead, Arsenic, and Mercury, have found their way into fish and shellfish.

Cadmium and Lead can significantly impede or interfere with the absorption of other Minerals. Cadmium can cause kidney damage, and lead can impair brain development.

Arsenic is believed to increase the risk of cancer.

Mercury, which has been consistently been found in large fish, particularly swordfish, king mackerel, tilefish, and shark, damages nerve cells. Because Mercury is especially damaging during prenatal development, pregnant women are advised to avoid certain types of fish and limit their consumption of others

Bio-Accumulation

Chemicals used in agricultural production and industrial wastes contaminate the environment and can find their way into the food supply. *How harmful these chemicals are depends on whether they persist in the environment and whether they accumulate in the organisms that consume them or can be broken down and excreted by those organisms.*

Some of these contaminants are eliminated from the environment quickly because they are able to be broken down by microorganisms or chemical reactions.

Others remain in the environment for very long periods, and when taken up by plants and small animals, they are not metabolized or excreted. When these plants or small animals are consumed by larger animals that are in turn eaten by still larger animals, the contaminants accumulate, reaching higher concentrations at each level of the food chain. This process is called **Bioaccumulation**.

Because the toxins are not eliminated from the body, the greater the amount consumed, the greater the amount present in the body. This un-natural process may be at the root-cause of several of the Health issues that are currently on the rise and that causes pre-mature death!

Bioaccumulation- The process by which compounds accumulate or build up in an organism faster than they can be broken down or excreted.

This is why it is paramount that if YOU haven't started your own Quality Food Supply = Garden......PLEASE STOP RIGHT NOW AND BEGIN!!!!!!!!

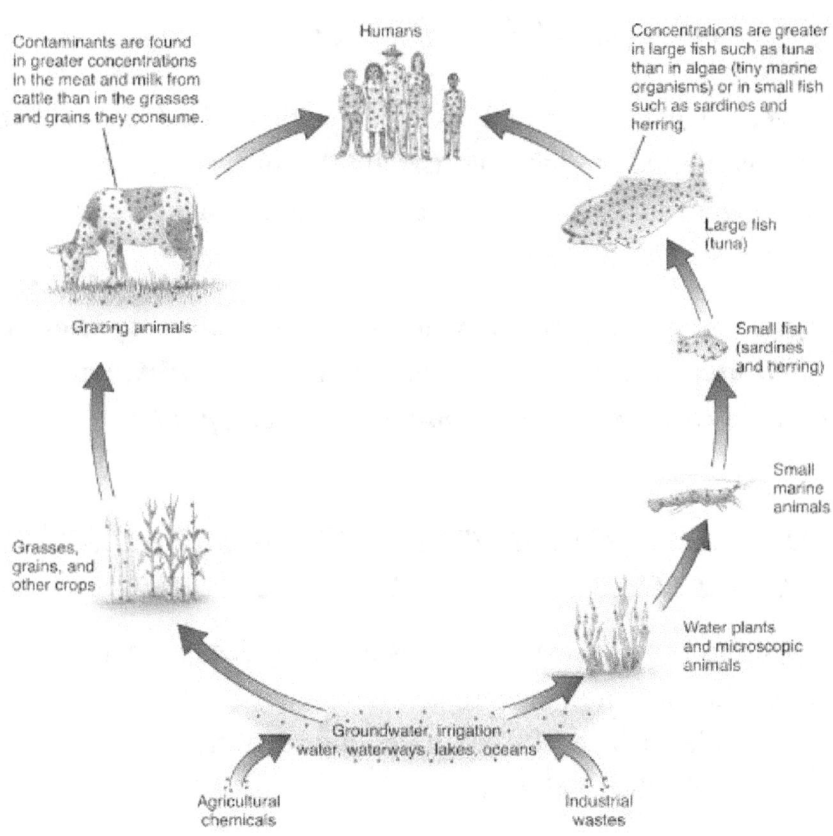

Contaminants are found in greater concentrations in the meat and milk from cattle than in the grasses and grains they consume.

Humans

Concentrations are greater in large fish such as tuna than in algae (tiny marine organisms) or in small fish such as sardines and herring.

Large fish (tuna)

Grazing animals

Small fish (sardines and herring)

Small marine animals

Grasses, grains, and other crops

Water plants and microscopic animals

Groundwater, irrigation water, waterways, lakes, oceans

Agricultural chemicals

Industrial wastes

Contamination Throughout Our Food Chain

Industrial pollutants and agricultural chemicals that contaminate the water supply enter the food chain and accumulate as they are passed through the chain.

Fat-soluble contaminants concentrate in body fat and cannot be excreted.

An animal that occupies a higher level in the food chain has higher concentrations of these contaminants because it consumes all the contaminants that have been eaten by organisms at lower feeding levels.

This science supports the fact as to WHY Humans ARE HERBIVORES…We eat directly and ONLY from the Primary Producers of Life Energy = Fruits and Veggies.

Pesticides: Risks & Benefits

Pesticides are used to prevent plant diseases and insect infestations. They are applied both to crops in the fields and to harvested produce in order to prevent spoilage and extend shelf life. Crops that are grown using pesticides generally produce higher yields and look more appealing because they have less insect damage.

Once they have been applied, however, pesticides can travel into water supplies, soil, and other parts of the environment. Because pesticides enter the environment, pesticide residues are found not only on the treated plants but also in meat, poultry, fish, and dairy products.

The potential risks of pesticides to consumers depend on the size, age, and health of the person who consumes the pesticides and on the type and amount consumed.

To protect public health and the environment, the types of pesticides that may be used on food crops, the frequency of their use, and the amount of residue that may remain when foods reach consumers are regulated. The EPA approves and registers pesticides that are used in food production and establishes **Tolerances**.

Pesticide Tolerances are the maximum amounts of pesticide residues that may remain in or on a food. *To establish tolerances that are safe for both children and adults, the EPA considers tests done in experimental animals and on cells growing in the laboratory, as well as the amount of the pesticide to which consumers are likely to be exposed.* ***Tolerances are then usually set at least 100 times lower than the highest dose that has no harmful effects in test animals.***

The FDA and the USDA monitor pesticide residues in foods. In general, pesticide residue levels in both domestic and imported foods have been found to be well below federally permitted limits.

These Tolerance levels that the FDA and USDA allow are broad, and intended to allow a specific number of people to become sick or die WITHOUT any repercussions to the manufacturer.

The FACT that they allow a Poisonous and TOXIC substance to be used on our food supply underscores the importance of GROWING YOUR OWN FOOD!

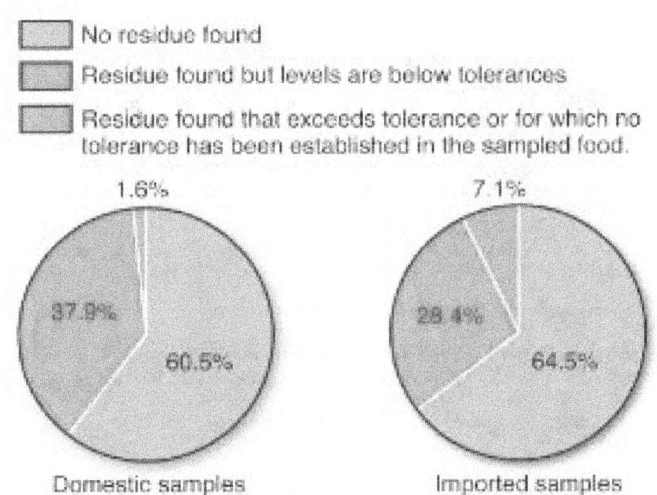

☐ No residue found

☐ Residue found but levels are below tolerances

☐ Residue found that exceeds tolerance or for which no tolerance has been established in the sampled food.

Domestic samples: 1.6%, 37.9%, 60.5%

Imported samples: 7.1%, 28.4%, 64.5%

In February of 2014, a California-based beef producer recalled almost nine million pounds of product that had never been inspected: The animals the meat came from were diseased. **A month earlier, the same company had been forced to recall 40 tons of uninspected beef.**

In the fall of 2013, two Colorado cantaloupe farmers pled guilty to criminal charges in connection with a Listeria outbreak that killed 33: They claimed they did not operate a melon-washing system properly.

THE ABOVE ARE EXAMPLES FROM BOTH ANIMAL AND PLANT BASED DISEASE OR DEATH……GROW YOUR OWN FOOD !!!!

Food-borne illnesses annually sicken 48 million Americans and kill 3000 of us. Even our water is sometimes threatened. *A third of a million West Virginians started out 2014 with contaminated tap water because of a chemical spill in the Elk River.*

Despite these frightening incidents, most food arrives in our homes safe and fit to eat, and it remains that way if we handle it properly.

The modern U.S. food supply is perhaps the safest in human history, but danger still lurks if adequate food-handling practices are not in place from farm or feedlot to table.

Agencies that monitor the food supply	
International Organizations	
Food and Agriculture Organization of the United Nations (FAO)	Promotes and shares knowledge in all aspects of food quality and safety and in all stages of food production: harvest, postharvest handling, storage, transport, processing, and distribution.
World Health Organization (WHO)	Develops international food safety policies, food inspection programs, and standards for hygienic food preparation; promotes technologies that improve food safety and consumer education about safe food practices. Works closely with the FAO.
Federal Organizations	
U.S. Food and Drug Administration (FDA)	Ensures the safety and quality of all foods sold across state lines with the exception of red meat, poultry, and egg products; inspects food processing plants; inspects imported foods with the exception of red meat, poultry, and egg products; sets standards for food composition; oversees use of drugs and feed in food-producing animals; enforces regulations for food labeling, food and color additives and food sanitation.
U.S. Department of Agriculture (USDA) Food Safety and Inspection Service (FSIS)	Enforces standards for the wholesomeness and quality of red meat, poultry, and egg products produced in the United States and imported from other countries. If an imported food is suspect, it can be tested for contamination and denied entry into the country.
U.S. Environmental Protection Agency (EPA)	Regulates pesticide levels and must approve all pesticides before they can be sold in the United States; establishes water quality standards.
National Marine Fisheries Service	Oversees the management of fisheries and fish harvesting; operates a voluntary program of inspection and grading of fish products.
National Oceanic and Atmospheric Administration (NOAA)	Oversees fish and seafood products. Its Seafood Inspection Program inspects and certifies fishing vessels, seafood processing plants, and retail facilities for compliance with federal sanitation standards.
Centers for Disease Control and Prevention (CDC)	Monitors and investigates the incidence and causes of food-borne illnesses.
State and Local Governments	
Oversee all food within their jurisdiction; also inspect restaurants, grocery stores, and other retail food establishments, as well as dairy farms and milk processing plants, grain mills, and food manufacturing plants within local jurisdictions.	

Cause & Effect

Each year, 1 in 6 Americans, or about 48 million people, get sick, 128,000 are hospitalized, and 3000 die from food-borne illnesses. Media coverage of outbreaks of food-borne illness on cruise ships, of deaths from *E. coli* infection, and of cows infected with mad cow disease have heightened public concern and led to the development of the National Food Safety Initiative. The goal of this initiative is to reduce the incidence of food-borne illness by improving food safety practices and policies throughout the United States.

Because food can be contaminated ***anywhere*** in the supply chain—from where it is grown to when it is served in your home—IT SHOULD MOTIVATE YOU TO IMMEDIATELY START YOUR OWN LIFE ENERGY (FOOD) SUPPLY!!!

food-borne illness - An illness caused by consumption of contaminated food.

Microbes - Microscopic organisms, or microorganisms, including bacteria, viruses, and fungi.

Whether or not you get sick from eating a contaminated food depends on how potent the contaminant is, how much of it you consume, and how often you consume it, as well as on your age, size, and health.

Some food contaminants cause harm even when minute amounts are consumed, and almost any substance can be toxic if a large enough amount of it is consumed.

How well a substance is absorbed and how it is metabolized by the body affect toxicity.

Dietary Factors and Nutritional Status can affect absorption. For example, Mercury, which is extremely toxic, is not absorbed well if the diet is high in Selenium, and Lead absorption is decreased by the presence of Iron and Calcium in the diet.

Contaminants that are stored in the body after being absorbed are more likely to be toxic because they accumulate over time, eventually causing symptoms of toxicity. Contaminants that are easily excreted from the body are less likely to cause toxicity.

An individual's size, overall health and nutritional status, and immune function affect his or her risk of food-borne illness. Infants and children are at greater risk than adults because their immune systems are immature and their small size means that a given amount of contaminant represents a greater amount per unit of body weight than it would in an adult.

Elderly people, people with AIDS, and those receiving chemotherapy or other immunosuppressant drugs are at increased risk because their immune systems may be compromised.

Pregnancy weakens the immune system, putting pregnant women and their unborn babies at risk.

Poor nutritional status and chronic conditions such as diabetes and kidney disease may decrease the body's ability to detoxify harmful substances.

Most cases of food-borne illness in the United States are caused by food that has been contaminated with **Pathogens**. The Pathogens that most commonly affect the food supply include bacteria, viruses, molds, and parasites.

A typical case of food-borne illness causes a short bout of flulike symptoms, including abdominal pain, nausea, diarrhea, and vomiting. However, more severe symptoms, such as kidney failure, arthritis, paralysis, miscarriage, and even death, sometimes occur.

1. **Farm** Crops can be contaminated with bacteria before they are even harvested. Good agricultural practices help minimize contamination during growing, harvesting, sorting, packing, and storage.

2. **Processing** Contamination of processing equipment can transfer microbes to food. To prevent contamination, processors must follow guidelines concerning cleanliness and training of workers; develop a protocol that anticipates how biological, chemical, or physical hazards are most likely to occur; and establish appropriate measures to prevent them from occurring.

3. **Transportation** During transport, poor sanitation and inadequate refrigeration can contaminate food and allow microbes to grow. Clean containers and vehicles, plus refrigeration, can prevent the growth of food-borne bacteria.

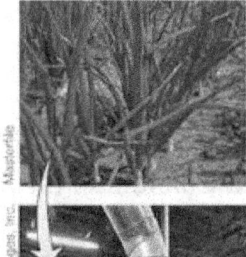
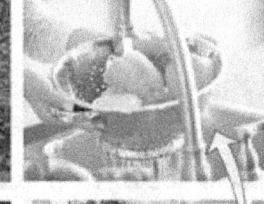
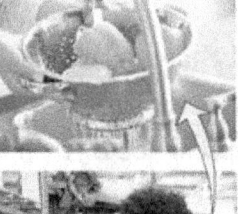
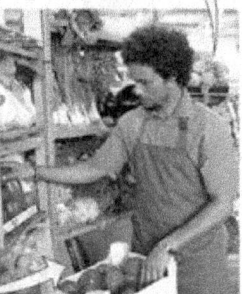

5. **Table** Even a safe food can be contaminated in the home. Consumers can prevent food-borne illness at their table by carefully washing hands and food preparation equipment, as well as by handling, storing, and preparing food properly.

4. **Retail** Food can become contaminated during handling or storage in grocery stores or during preparation in restaurants. The FDA's Food Code provides recommendations for the handling and service of food in an effort to help owners and employees at retail establishments prevent food-borne illness. Local health inspections ensure cleanliness and proper procedures.

Pathogen- A biological agent that causes disease.

Any food-borne illness caused by pathogens that multiply in the human body is called a **Food-Borne Infection**. Contracting a food-borne infection usually involves consumption of a large number of Pathogens that infect the body or produce Toxins within the body. Any food-borne illness caused by consuming a food that contains toxins produced by pathogens is referred to as **Food-Borne Intoxication**.

Even food that contains only a *few* Pathogens can cause Food-Borne Intoxication if the pathogens have produced enough Toxin.

Sean Ali
Understanding Our Human Energy System!

Avoiding food-borne illness—both infection and intoxication—requires knowing how to handle and store food in ways that will prevent contamination and prevent or minimize the growth of pathogens that may already be present in the food.

Even a food that is contaminated with pathogens can be safe if it is prepared in a manner that destroys any pathogens or toxins that are present.

Bacteria in Food

Bacteria are present in the soil, on our skin, on most surfaces in our homes, and in the food we eat. Most are harmless, some are beneficial, and a few are pathogenic, causing food-borne infection or intoxication.

Salmonella is the most common cause of bacterial food-borne illness in the United States. Although poultry and eggs are the foods most often contaminated with *Salmonella*, it has also been found in a variety of foods ranging from peanut butter, ground meat, fruits, and vegetables to processed foods such as frozen pot pies. Because *Salmonella* is killed by heat, foods that are likely to be contaminated should be cooked thoroughly.

Campylobacter Jejuni is a leading cause of acute bacterial diarrhea in the United States, affecting about 845,000 people annually. Common sources are undercooked chicken, unpasteurized milk, cheeses made from unpasteurized milk, and untreated water.

A sampling of raw chicken from supermarkets from 2005 to 2011 found that about 40% of samples were contaminated with *Campylobacter*. This organism grows slowly in cold temperatures and is killed by heat, so careful storage and thorough cooking are key to preventing infection.

Escherichia coli, commonly called *E. coli*, is a bacterium that inhabits the gastrointestinal tracts of humans and other animals. It comes into contact with food through fecal contamination of water or unsanitary handling of food.

Some strains of *E. coli* are harmless, but others can cause serious food-borne infection. ***One strain of E. coli, found in water contaminated by human or animal feces, is the cause of "travelers' diarrhea."***

Another strain, *E. coli* O157:H7, produces a toxin in the body that causes abdominal pain, bloody diarrhea, and in severe cases a form of kidney failure called **hemolytic-uremic syndrome**, which can be fatal.

E. coli O157:H7 entered the public spotlight in 1993, when it led to the deaths of several children who had consumed undercooked, contaminated hamburgers from a fast-food restaurant. Thorough cooking of the hamburgers would have killed the bacteria that caused these deaths.

 E. coli can also contaminate produce such as lettuce, spinach, and green onions and cause illness if the produce is eaten raw. In 2013, *E. coli* contamination of ready-to-eat salads sickened people in four states.

This is WHY we MUST grow our own Food. Food is our Energy Source, and we can only grow and develop as our food is grown and developed.

In 2011, infected bologna, another food that we don't typically cook, sickened people in five different states. In addition to concerns about *E. coli* O157:H7 in our meat and produce, a new, even more deadly strain of *E. coli* emerged in Europe in 2011, ultimately sickening more than 4000 people in 16 countries.

Although food-borne *Listeria monocytogenes* sickens fewer people than *Salmonella* or *Campylobacter*, this bacterium is one of the leading causes of death from food-borne illness, with a fatality rate of 21%. Almost all *Listeria* infections occur in people in high-risk groups, such as pregnant women, children, elderly people, and people with compromised immune systems.

Listeria is ubiquitous in the environment and can survive and grow at refrigerator temperatures. ***Because it can grow at cool temperatures, this bacterium can infect ready-to-eat foods such as hot dogs, lunch meats, smoked fish, and cheeses even if they have been kept properly refrigerated***. To prevent infection, ready-to-eat meats should be heated to the steaming point, and unpasteurized dairy products should be avoided.

Vibrio bacteria can cause illness when contaminated seafood is eaten. *Vibrio* infection causes gastrointestinal upset but can be deadly in people with compromised immune systems.

Vibrio Parahaemolyticus sickens about 45,000 people per year. Another species, *Vibrio Vulnificus*, infects fewer people but is more often fatal.

The most common way in which people become infected is by eating raw or undercooked shellfish, particularly oysters.

Vibrio bacteria grow in warm seawater. The incidence of *Vibrio* infection is higher during the summer months, when warm water favors growth.

Bacterial Food-Borne Intoxication

Staphylococcus aureus is a common cause of bacterial food-borne intoxication. These bacteria live in human nasal passages and can be transferred to food through coughing or sneezing. They can then grow on the food, producing a toxin that causes vomiting soon after ingestion.

Another cause of food-borne intoxication is the bacterium Clostridium perfringens. It is often called the Cafeteria Germ because it grows in foods that are stored in large containers like those used in cafeterias*.** Little oxygen gets to the food at the center of a large container, thus providing an excellent growth environment for bacteria such as these, which thrive in low-oxygen environments. ***C. Perfringens are difficult to kill because they form heat-resistant Spore.

Spores are a stage of bacterial life that remains dormant until environmental conditions favor their growth. *C. perfringens* may cause illness through both infection and intoxication.

The deadliest of all bacterial food toxins is produced by *Clostridium botulinum*. ***Heat-resistant spores of C. Botulinum are found in soil, water, and the intestinal tracts of animals***.

Growing our own food helps to eliminate the potential soil or water contamination and eating as a Human = HERBIVORE, eliminates poisoning from animal meats….because You can't cook Botulism out of food.

The toxin is produced when the spores begin to grow and develop. When consumed, the toxin blocks nerve function, resulting in vomiting, abdominal pain, double vision, and paralysis that leads to respiratory failure.

If untreated, **Botulism** is often fatal, but modern detection methods and rapid administration of antitoxin have reduced mortality rates.

C. b\Botulinum grows in low-oxygen, low-acid conditions, so improperly canned foods and foods such as potatoes or stew that are held in large containers where there is little exposure to oxygen provide optimal conditions for botulism spores to germinate.

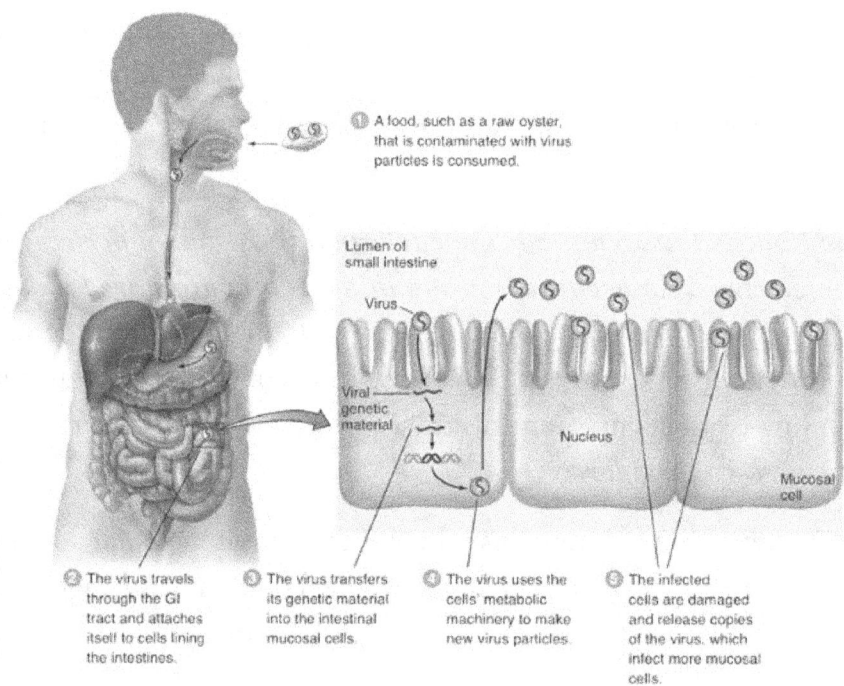

Noroviruses are a group of viruses that cause gastroenteritis, or what we commonly call "stomach flu." These viruses are the leading cause of food-borne illness in the United States, sickening 5.5 million people per year.

Norovirus illness is contracted either by eating food that is contaminated with the virus or by touching a contaminated surface and then putting your fingers in your mouth.

Shellfish can be contaminated with norovirus if the water in which they live is polluted with human or animal feces.

Cooking destroys noroviruses, so water and uncooked foods such as leafy vegetables, fruits, and nuts are the most common causes of norovirus food-borne illness. Most outbreaks are caused by food contaminated during preparation and service; one study found that infected food handlers may have contributed to 82% of the outbreaks examined. *This is WHY we must grow, prepare and cook our own Food....Food is our way of extending our Lifespan and simultaneously improving the Quality of our Lives!*

Norovirus infection can be spread from one infected person to another, so it spreads swiftly where many people congregate in a small area. You may have heard of it as a cause of food-borne illness aboard cruise ships.

These outbreaks make headlines, but norovirus outbreaks are just as likely in nursing homes, restaurants, hotels, and dormitories as they are aboard cruise ships.

Hepatitis A is another viral infection that can be contracted from food or water that is contaminated with fecal matter. Hepatitis A infection causes liver inflammation, jaundice, fever, nausea, fatigue, and abdominal pain. The infection can require a recovery period of several months, but it does not require treatment and does not cause permanent liver damage. Hepatitis in drinking water is destroyed by chlorination. Cooking destroys the virus in food, and good sanitation can prevent its spread. There is a vaccine that is advertised to protect against Hepatitis A infection that is available.

Moldy Foods

There are many types of **Mold** that grows on foods such as bread, cheese, and fruit. Under certain conditions, these Molds produce toxins. More than 250 different mold Toxins have been identified. *Cooking and freezing stop mold growth but do not destroy toxins that have already been produced. If a food is moldy, it should be discarded, the area where it was stored should be cleaned, and neighboring foods should be checked to see if they have also become contaminated.*

Mold- Multi-cellular Fungi that form filamentous branching growths.

Parasites in Food

Some **Parasites** are microscopic single-celled animals, and others manifest as worms that become large enough to be seen with the naked eye. ***Parasites that can be transmitted through consumption of contaminated food and water cause food-borne illness***.

Cryptosporidium Parvum is another single-celled parasite that causes diarrhea. It is commonly contracted from and spread by contaminated water, and the life stage of the parasite that causes infection is resistant to chlorine.

Parasite- An Organism that lives at the expense of another.

Trichinella Spiralis is a Parasite that is found in raw and undercooked pork and game meats. Once ingested, these small, wormlike organisms find their way to the muscles, where they grow, causing flulike symptoms.

Fish are another common source of parasitic infections because they carry the larvae of parasites such as roundworms, flatworms, flukes, and tapeworms (Figure Below). ***As the popularity of eating raw fish has increased, so has the incidence of parasitic infections from fish***. Parasites, including those in fish, are killed by thorough cooking. When consuming raw fish, parasitic infections can be avoided by eating fish that has been frozen.

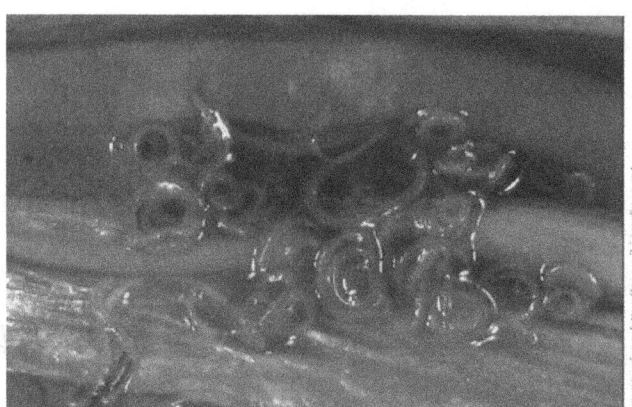

Image from http://en.wikipedia.org/wiki/File:Anisakids.jpg

Prions in Food

The strangest and scariest, yet rarest, food-borne illness is caused not by a microbe but by a protein, called a **prion**, that has folded improperly. Abnormal prions are believed to be the cause of mad cow disease, or **bovine spongiform encephalopathy (BSE)**, a deadly degenerative neurological disease that affects cattle. The human form of this disease is **variant Creutzfeldt-Jakob Disease (vCJD)**. *People are believed to contract it by eating tissue from a cow infected with BSE.* <u>*Symptoms of vCJD begin as mood swings and numbness and within about 14 months progress to dementia and death.*</u>

Prion - A pathogenic Protein that is the cause of degenerative brain diseases called spongiform encephalopathies. Prion is short for *Proteinaceous Infectious Particle.*

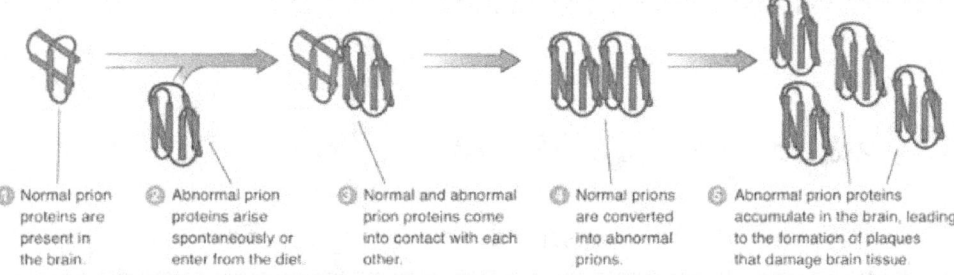

1. Normal prion proteins are present in the brain.
2. Abnormal prion proteins arise spontaneously or enter from the diet.
3. Normal and abnormal prion proteins come into contact with each other.
4. Normal prions are converted into abnormal prions.
5. Abnormal prion proteins accumulate in the brain, leading to the formation of plaques that damage brain tissue

How Prions Multiply

The abnormal prions that cause BSE differ from normal proteins in the way they are folded—that is, in their three-dimensional structure. <u>*When the improperly folded form of a prion is introduced into the brain after a person has eaten contaminated tissue, it can reproduce by corrupting neighboring proteins, essentially changing their shape so that they, too, become abnormal prions*</u>. Because the abnormal prions are not degraded normally, they accumulate and form clumps called plaques. These plaques cause deadly nervous tissue damage.

The understanding of Prions lends further support to the FACT that Humans ARE HERBIVORES……And that a majority of the dis-eases that Humans suffer are caused by eating other-than-Human foods.

What Bug Has You Down?

There are certainly a wide variety of food-borne pathogens that can make you sick. Recent improvements in governmental outbreak surveillance, attentiveness by health-care professionals, and testing frequency and accuracy have made it possible to identify even more cases of food-borne illness than was possible a few years ago.

Despite the added attention, data that measures trends in food-borne disease indicate that there has not been much progress in reducing food-borne infections; the incidence of infection with nine key pathogens was not significantly different in 2013 than in 2006–2008.

Public awareness of the problem and education on how to handle food safely can help reduce the incidence of food-borne illness in the future.

Preventing Microbial Food-Borne Illness

Microbes in food multiply when they are presented with the right conditions for growth. Choosing food carefully can help reduce the risk of microbial food-borne illness by minimizing the number of food-borne pathogens brought into the home. Once at home, preparing food in a clean kitchen reduces **Cross-Contamination**.

Storing food at refrigerator or freezer temperatures either limits or stops microbial growth. Heating foods to the recommended temperature kills microbes and destroys toxins.

Foods that are served cold should be kept cold until they are served. Frozen foods should be kept frozen and then thawed in the refrigerator or microwave before cooking, not thawed at room temperature, which favors microbial growth.

Cooked food should be handled with care and kept hot until it is served and chilled quickly before storage.

<u>When in doubt about the safety of a food, throw it out.</u>

**Growing our own food so we can go from Garden to Table is the Best and ONLY wat to ensure Total Food Safety!**

**We can ONLY grow and develop as our food is grown and developed…..do YOU know WHO is Growing the Food YOU eat??**

**When we grow our own food, we KNOW what is being used on it for it to produce and we KNOW it is being Harvested = Maximum Quality and Quantity of Life Energy**!

Summary of bacterial, viral, and parasitic food-borne illnesses				
Microbe	Sources	Symptoms	Onset (time after consumption)	Duration
Bacteria				
Campylobacter jejuni	Unpasteurized milk, untreated water, undercooked meat and poultry	Fever, headache, diarrhea, abdominal pain	2–5 days	2–10 days
Clostridium botulinum	Improperly canned foods, deep-dish casseroles, honey	Lassitude, weakness, vertigo, respiratory failure, paralysis	18–36 hours	10 days or longer (must administer antitoxin)
Clostridium perfringens	Fecal contamination, deep-dish casseroles	Nausea, diarrhea, abdominal pain	about 16 hours	12–24 hours
Escherichia coli O157:H7	Fecal contamination, undercooked ground beef	Abdominal pain, bloody diarrhea, kidney failure	1–9 days	2–9 days in uncomplicated cases
Listeria monocytogenes	Raw milk products; soft ripened cheeses; deli meats and cold cuts; raw and undercooked poultry; meats; raw and smoked fish; raw vegetables	Fever, headache, stiff neck, chills, nausea, vomiting. May cause spontaneous abortion or stillbirth in pregnant women and meningitis and blood infections in the fetus.	Hours to weeks	Days to weeks
Salmonella	Fecal contamination; raw or undercooked eggs and meat, especially poultry; contaminated produce	Nausea, abdominal pain, diarrhea, headache, fever	6–72 hours	4–7 days
Shigella	Fecal contamination of foods, especially salads such as chicken, tuna, shrimp, and potato salads	Diarrhea, abdominal pain, fever, vomiting	8–50 hours	5–7 days
Staphylococcus aureus	Human contamination from coughs and sneezes; eggs, meat, potato and macaroni salads	Severe nausea, vomiting, diarrhea	1–7 hours	Hours–1 day
Vibrio parahaemolyticus	Raw seafood from contaminated water	Cramps, diarrhea, fever, nausea, vomiting	4–90 hours	2–6 days
Yersinia enterocolitica	Pork, unpasteurized milk, and oysters	Diarrhea, vomiting, fever, abdominal pain; often mistaken for appendicitis	1–11 days	A few days – 3 weeks
Viruses				
Hepatitis A	Human fecal contamination of food or water, raw shellfish	Jaundice, liver inflammation, fatigue, fever, nausea, anorexia, abdominal discomfort	15–50 days	1–2 weeks to several months
Norovirus	Fecal contamination of water or foods, especially shellfish and salad ingredients	Diarrhea, nausea, vomiting	24–48 hours	12–60 hours
Parasites				
Anisakis simplex	Raw fish	Severe abdominal pain	24 hours–2 weeks	3 weeks
Cryptosporidium parvum	Fecal contamination of food or water	Severe watery diarrhea	7–10 days	2–14 days, but may become chronic
Giardia lamblia	Fecal contamination of water and uncooked foods	Diarrhea, abdominal pain, gas, anorexia, nausea, vomiting	1–2 weeks	2–6 weeks, but may be chronic
Toxoplasma gondii	Meat, primarily pork	Toxoplasmosis (can cause central nervous system disorders, flulike symptoms, and birth defects in the offspring of women exposed during pregnancy; see Chapter 11)	5–23 days	Several weeks, but may become chronic
Trichinella spiralis	Undercooked pork, game meat	Muscle weakness, flulike symptoms	1–4 weeks	Several weeks

*Chapter Twelve ...

Energy Assessment*

****

Nutritional Status

Nutritional Status can be established by measuring indicators of Nutrient Stores. Variations of Nutrient Stores result in changes in Nutritional Status when the nutrient needs and nutrient use are increased or alterations in Nutrient Intake occur. Inadequacy or excess of a particular nutrient produces Physiologic alteration in the body.

Careful attention to physical signs of possible malnutrition provides an added dimension to the overall assessment of general nutritional status.

EXTENT OF BODY RESERVES OF NUTRIENTS

NUTRIENT	TIME REQUIRED TO DEPLETE RESERVES IN WELL-NOURISHED INDIVIDUALS
Amino acids	Several hours
Carbohydrate	13 hours
Sodium	2-3 days
Water	4 days
Zinc	5 days
Fat	20-40 days
Thiamin	30-60 days
Vitamin C	60-120 days
Niacin	60-180 days
Riboflavin	60-180 days
Vitamin A	90-365 days
Iron	125 days (women), 750 days (men)
Iodine	1000 days
Calcium	2500 days

Nutrition Assessment

Nutrition assessment is "a systematic approach to collect, record, and interpret relevant data from patients, clients, family members, caregivers and other individuals and groups. It is an ongoing, dynamic process that involves initial data collection as well as continual reassessment and analysis of the patient's/client's status compared to specified criteria."

The fundamental purpose of nutrition assessment in general clinical practice is to determine the following three factors:

1. Overall nutritional status of the patient

2. Current health care needs—physical, psychosocial, and personal.

3. Related factors influencing these needs in the person's current life situation

Step 1: Nutrition Assessment

Techniques such as those outlined in the chapter are used to systematically obtain information necessary to determine or reassess whether or not a nutrition problem (or diagnosis) exists. If so, then the problem is diagnosed using a PES (Problem, Etiology, Signs and Symptoms) statement in step 2 of the NCP.

Step 2: Nutrition Diagnosis

Before nutrition intervention can take place, the nutrition problem (or problems) must be identified. This is accomplished with the nutrition diagnosis. Standardized language is used to make the nutrition diagnosis clear to other nutrition and health care professionals. When the nutrition problem has been identified, it is labeled with a specific, standardized diagnostic term.

The nutrition diagnosis statement or PES statement is organized in three distinct parts: (1) the Problem (P);

(2) the Etiology, or cause, of the problem (E); and

3) the Signs and Symptoms associated with the problem (S).

Typically, nutrition diagnoses fall into three categories or domains:

1. Intake

2. Clinical

3. Behavioral-environmental

The following is an example of how a nutrition diagnosis is written:

A disordered eating pattern is *related to* harmful beliefs about food and nutrition *as evidenced by* the reported use of laxatives after meals and statements that calories are not absorbed when laxatives are used.

Step 3: Nutrition Intervention

Intervention begins once the nutritional diagnosis is identified. It is generally aimed at the Etiology (E) of the nutrition diagnosis and is directed at reducing or eradicating effects of the Signs and Symptoms (S).

Nutrition interventions are intended to modify a nutrition-related problem and comprise two interconnected components: (1) Planning and (2) Implementation.

Nutrition Diagnoses are prioritized in the planning component, whereby implementation is the "Action Phase."

The plan is communicated and carried out, data continue to be collected, and nutrition interventions are revised as necessary. *Four categories or domains of nutrition intervention have been identified*:

1. Food and/or nutrient delivery

2. Nutrition education

3. Nutrition counseling

4. Coordination of care

Step 4: Nutrition Monitoring and Evaluation

The point of this step in the NCP is to measure improvement made by the patient in meeting nutrition care goals. Patients' progress is examined by determining if the nutrition intervention is being executed and by providing evidence that the intervention _is_ or _is not_ altering the patients' nutritional status.

**Nutrition monitoring and evaluation terms are organized into four categories or domains**:

1. Food- and nutrition-related history

2. Biochemical data, medical tests, and procedures

3. Anthropometric measurements

4. Nutrition-focused physical findings

In summary, the NCP allows for continuous treatment alteration. As patients' conditions change, so do diagnoses, plans, and interventions. If patients do not respond to interventions, then new interventions can be developed for them. However, it is important to remember that any and all nutrition interventions should be planned in consultation with patients, as well as with their caregivers or significant others

Clinical Signs of Nutritional Status

Careful attention to physical signs of possible malnutrition provides an added dimension to the overall assessment of general nutritional status. A guide for a general examination of such signs is given in the Table below.

Page | 190

AREA OF CONCERN	POSSIBLE DEFICIENCY	POSSIBLE EXCESS
Hair		
Dull, dry, brittle	Pro	
Easily plucked (with no pain)	Pro	
Hair loss	Pro, Zn, biotin	Vit A
Flag sign (loss of hair pigment in strips around head)	Pro, Cu	
Head & Neck		
Bulging fontanel (infants)		Vit A
Headache		Vit A, D
Epistaxis (nosebleed)	Vit K	
Thyroid enlargement	Iodine	
Eyes		
Conjunctival and corneal xerosis (dryness)	Vit A	
Pale conjunctiva	Fe	
Blue sclerae	Fe	
Corneal vascularization	Vit B_2	

AREA OF CONCERN	POSSIBLE DEFICIENCY	POSSIBLE EXCESS
Mouth		
Cheilosis/Angular Stomatitis (lesions at corners mouth)	Vit B_2	
Glossitis (red, sore tongue)	Niacin, folate, vit B_{12}, and other B vit	
Gingivitis (inflamed gums)	Vit C	
Hypogeusia, dysgeusia (distorted & poor sense of taste)	Zn	
Dental caries	Fluoride	
Mottling of teeth		Fluoride
Atrophy of papillae on tongue	Fe, B vit	
Skin		
Dry, scaly	Vit A, Zn, EFAs	Vit A
Follicular hyperkeratosis (resembles gooseflesh)	Vit A, EFAs, B vit	
Eczematous lesions	Zn	
Petechiae, ecchymoses	Vit C, K	
Nasolabial seborrhea (greasy, scaly areas between nose and lip)	Niacin, vit B_{12}, B_6	
Darkening and peeling of skin in areas exposed to sun	Niacin	
Poor wound healing	Pro, Zn, vit C	
Nails		
Spoon-shaped nails	Fe	
Brittle, fragile	Pro	

AREA OF CONCERN	POSSIBLE DEFICIENCY	POSSIBLE EXCESS

Heart

AREA OF CONCERN	POSSIBLE DEFICIENCY	POSSIBLE EXCESS
Enlargement, tachycardia, failure	Vit B_1	
Small heart	Energy	
Sudden failure, death	Se	
Arrhythmia	Mg, K, Se	
Hypertension	Ca, K	

Abdomen

AREA OF CONCERN	POSSIBLE DEFICIENCY	POSSIBLE EXCESS
Hepatomegaly	Pro	Vit A
Ascites	Pro	

Musculoskeletal Extremities

AREA OF CONCERN	POSSIBLE DEFICIENCY	POSSIBLE EXCESS
Muscle wasting (especially temporal area)	Energy	
Edema	Pro, vit B_1	
Calf tenderness	Vit B_1 or C, biotoin, Se	
Beading of ribs, or "rachitic rosary" (child)	Vit C, D	
Bone and joint tenderness	Vit C, D, Ca, P	
Knock-knee, bowed legs, fragile bones	Vit D, Ca, P, Cu	

Neurologic

AREA OF CONCERN	POSSIBLE DEFICIENCY	POSSIBLE EXCESS
Paresthesias (pain/ tingling & altered sensation in extremities)	Vit B_1, B_6, B_{12}, biotin	
Weakness	Vit C, B_1, B_6, B_{12}, energy	

Page | 193

AREA OF CONCERN	POSSIBLE DEFICIENCY	POSSIBLE EXCESS
Ataxia, decreased position and vibratory senses	Vit B_1, B_{12}	
Tremor	Mg	
Decreased tendon reflexes	Vit B_1	
Confabulation, disorientation	Vit B_1, B_{12}	
Drowsiness, lethargy	Vit B_1	Vit A, D
Depression	Vit B_1, biotin, B_{12}	

Ca, Calcium; *Cu,* copper; *EFAs,* essential fatty acids; *Fe,* iron; *K,* potassium, *Mg,* magnesium; *Na,* sodium; *P,* phosphorus; *Pro,* protein; *Se,* selenium; *Vit,* vitamin(s); *Zn,* zinc.

Principles of a nutrition therapy will be based on modifications of nutritional components of the normal diet as a particular disease condition may require. These changes may include the following types of modifications:

• *Nutrients:* modification of one or more of the basic nutrients—protein, carbohydrate, fat, minerals, and vitamins

• *Energy:* modification in energy value as expressed in kilocalories (kcalories or kcal)

• *Texture:* modification in texture or seasoning, such as liquid or low residue

RECOMMENDED DIETARY INTAKES (RDIS) USED TO ESTABLISH DAILY VALUES

Recommended Dietary Intakes (RDIs)* Used to Establish Daily Values

Source: USDA Food Labeling Guide. Available online at http://www.cfsan.fda.gov/~dms/2lg-xf.htm

Vitamins and Minerals	Units of Measurement	Adults and Children 4 or more Years of Age	Infants	Children Under 4 Years of Age	Pregnant or Lactating Women
Vitamin A	International Units†	5000 (1000 µg)	1500	2500	8000
Vitamin D	International Units†	400 (10 µg)	400	400	400
Vitamin E	International Units†	30 (10 µg)	5	10	30
Vitamin C	Milligrams	60	35	40	60
Folic acid	Micrograms	400	0.1	0.2	0.8
Thiamin	Milligrams	1.5	0.5	0.7	1.7
Riboflavin	Milligrams	1.7	0.6	0.8	2.0
Niacin	Milligrams	20	8	9	20
Vitamin B_6	Milligrams	2.0	0.4	0.7	2.5
Vitamin B_{12}	Micrograms	6.0	2	3	8
Biotin	Micrograms	300	0.05	0.15	0.30
Pantothenic acid	Milligrams	10	3	5	10
Calcium	Milligrams	1000	0.6	0.8	1.3
Phosphorous	Milligrams	1000	0.5	0.8	1.3
Iodine	Micrograms	150	45	70	150
Iron	Milligrams	18	15	10	18
Magnesium	Milligrams	400	70	200	450
Copper	Milligrams	2.0	0.6	1.0	2.0
Zinc	Milligrams	15	5	8	15
Vitamin K	Micrograms	80	‡	‡	‡
Chromium	Micrograms	120	—	—	—
Selenium	Micrograms	70	—	—	—
Molybdenum	Micrograms	75	—	—	—
Manganese	Milligrams	2	—	—	—
Chloride	Milligrams	3400	—	—	—

*Based on National Academy of Sciences' 1968 Recommended Dietary Allowances.

†The RDIs for fat-soluble vitamins are expressed in International Units (IU). Values that are approximately equivalent in micrograms are given in parentheses.

‡No values yet established for vitamin K, chromium, selenium, molybdenum, manganese, or chloride for this population.

Chapter Thirteen...

*Dangers of Supplements**

****

Citius, Altius, Fortius—faster, higher, stronger—is the motto of the Olympic Games. For as long as there have been competitions, athletes have yearned for anything that would give them a competitive edge. *Everything from bee pollen and high-dose vitamins to ancient herbs and hormones has been used as an **Ergogenic Aid**.*

Ergogenic Aid A substance, an appliance, or a procedure that improves athletic performance.

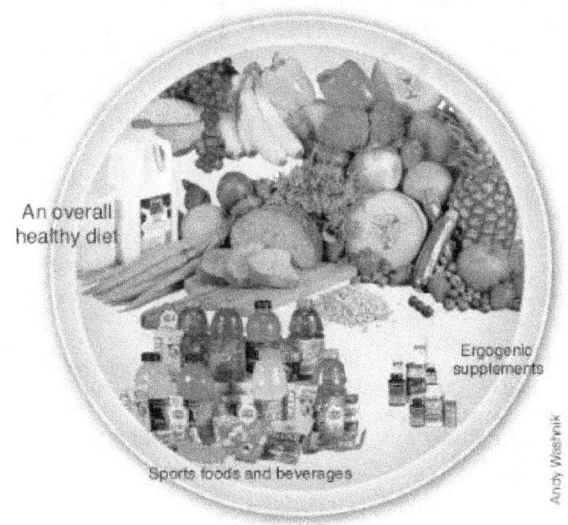

Athletes are willing to go to great lengths to improve performance and are therefore susceptible to the lures of Ergogenic supplements. Many of the Vitamins, Minerals, and other substances in these supplements are involved in providing energy for exercise or promoting recovery from exercise.

Most supplements do not improve athletic performance, and the few that do have a small effect compared to the benefits of an overall healthy diet.

When considering whether to use an ergogenic supplement or any other type of supplement, an individual risk–benefit analysis should be used to determine whether the supplement is appropriate for you.

Practice Safety with Dietary Supplements

When it comes to purchasing dietary supplements, Vasilios Frankos, Ph.D., Director of FDA's Division of Dietary Supplement Programs, offers this advice: "Be savvy!"

Today's dietary supplements are not only vitamins and minerals. "They also include other less familiar substances such as herbals, botanicals, amino acids, and enzymes," Frankos says. "Check with your health care providers before combining or substituting them with other foods or medicines." Frankos adds, "Do not self-diagnose any health condition. Work with your health care providers to determine how best to achieve optimal health."

Consider the following tips before buying a dietary supplement:
- Think twice about chasing the latest headline. Sound health advice is generally based on research over time, not a single study touted by the media. Be wary of results claiming a "quick fix" that departs from scientific research and established dietary guidance.
- More may not be better. Some products can be harmful when consumed in high amounts, for a long time, or in combination with certain other substances.
- Learn to spot false claims. If something sounds too good to be true, it probably is. Examples of false claims on product labels include:
  - Quick and effective "cure-all"
  - Can treat or cure disease
  - "Totally safe," "all natural," and has "definitely no side effects"

Other red flags include claims about limited availability, offers of "no-risk, money-back guarantees," and requirements for advance payment.

"Also ask yourself, 'Is the product worth the money!'" Frankos advises. "Resist the pressure to buy a product or treatment on the spot. Some supplement products may be expensive or may not provide the benefit you expect. For example, excessive amounts of water-soluble vitamins, like vitamins C and B, are not used by the body and are eliminated in the urine."

Vitamin and Mineral Supplements

Many of the promises made to athletes about the benefits of Vitamin and Mineral Supplements are extrapolated from the bio-chemical functions of these Micronutrients.

For example, B Vitamins are promoted to enhance ATP production because of their roles in muscle energy metabolism. Vitamin B_6, vitamin B_{12}, and Folic Acid are promoted for Aerobic exercise because they are involved in the transport of Oxygen to exercising muscles.

These vitamins are indeed needed for energy metabolism, and a deficiency of one or more of them will interfere with ATP production and impair athletic performance.

But providing more than the recommended amount does not deliver more oxygen to the muscles, cause more ATP to be produced, or enhance athletic performance.

How Vitamins are Regulated
Vitamin products are regulated by FDA as "Dietary Supplements." The law defines dietary supplements, in part, as products taken by mouth that contain a "dietary ingredient" intended to supplement the diet.

Listed in the "dietary ingredient" category are not only vitamins, but minerals, botanicals products, amino acids, and substances such as enzymes, microbial probiotics, and metabolites. Dietary supplements can also be extracts or concentrates, and may be found in many forms. The Dietary Supplement Health and Education Act of 1994 requires that all such products be labeled as dietary supplements.

In June 2007, FDA established dietary supplement "current Good Manufacturing Practice" (cGMP) regulations requiring that manufacturers evaluate their products through testing identity, purity, strength, and composition.

Supplements of Vitamin E, Vitamin C, and Selenium are promoted to athletes because of their antioxidant functions. As discussed earlier, exercise increases Oxidative processes and therefore increases the production of free-radicals, which cause Cellular damage and have been associated with fatigue. ***However, antioxidant supplements have not been found to improve performance.***

Supplements of Chromium (Chromium Picolinate) and Vanadium (Vanadyl Sulfate) are marketed to increase lean body mass and decrease body fat.

Chromium is needed for Insulin action, and the Insulin promotes Protein synthesis. However, studies have not consistently demonstrated that supplemental Chromium has any effect on muscle strength, body composition, or other aspects of health

Supplements to Build Muscle

Protein supplements are often marketed to athletes with the *promise* of enhancing muscle growth or improving performance. Adequate Protein is necessary for muscle growth, but consuming *extra* Protein, either as food or as supplements, ***does not increase muscle growth or strength***.

Muscles enlarge in response to exercise stress. The Protein provided by expensive supplements will ***not*** meet an athlete's needs any better than the Protein found in a balanced diet. If an athlete's diet provides enough energy, it usually provides enough Protein, without a supplement.

Anabolic steroids accelerate Protein Synthesis. When taken in conjunction with exercise and an adequate diet, they cause increases in muscle size and strength. ***However, they have extremely dangerous side effects***.

The Anabolic Steroid Control Act of 1990 made possession of anabolic steroids without a prescription illegal. The act was amended in 2004 to include **Steroid Precursors**, which are compounds that can be converted into steroid hormones in the body. The best known of these is androstenedione, often referred to as "andro." It was launched to public prominence when professional baseball player Mark McGwire announced his use of it during the 1998 major league baseball season, when he hit 70 home runs, breaking the league's single-season home-run record. Contrary to marketing claims, the use of Andro or other steroid precursors has not been found to increase testosterone levels or produce any ergogenic effects, and they may cause some of the same side effects as anabolic steroids.

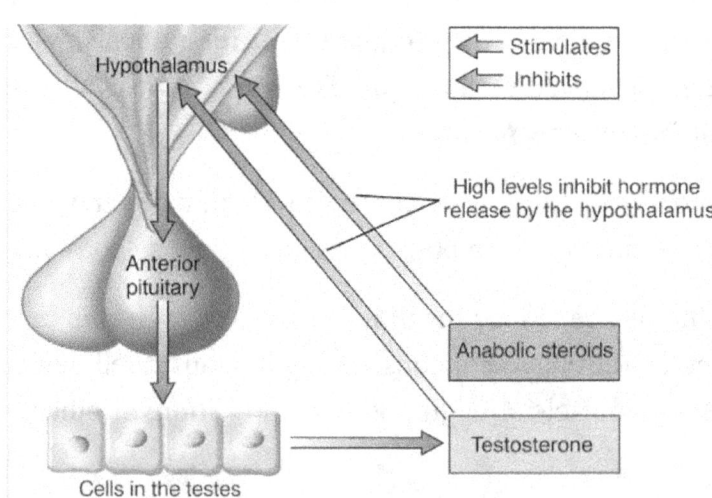

Anabolic Steroids- Synthetic fat-soluble hormones that mimic testosterone and are used to increase muscle strength and mass.

When testosterone levels are low, the Hypothalamus releases a Hormone that stimulates the Anterior Pituitary to secrete a hormone that increases the production of Testosterone by the Testes. ***High levels of either natural or synthetic testosterone inhibit the release of the stimulatory hormone from the hypothalamus, shutting down the synthesis of natural testosterone.***

A scientist sees that these are ***not*** the only effects that Anabolic Steroids have. ***These drugs make the body think natural testosterone is being produced, and therefore, as shown in the diagram, the body shuts down its own testosterone production***.

Natural testosterone stimulates and maintains the male sexual organs and promotes the development of bones and muscles and the growth of skin and hair. The Synthetic Testosterone in anabolic steroids has a greater effect on muscle, bone, skin, and hair than it does on sexual organs. ***<u>Without natural testosterone, the sexual organs are not maintained; this leads to shrinkage of the testicles and a decrease in sperm production</u>***.

Growth Hormone is another Hormone used to increase Muscle Protein Synthesis. Despite this physiological effect, however, it has not been shown to enhance muscle strength, power, or aerobic exercise capacity, but there is evidence that it improves anaerobic exercise capacity.

 Prolonged use of growth hormone can cause heart dysfunction, high blood pressure, and excessive growth of some body parts, such as hands, feet, and facial features. Growth hormone is on the World Anti-Doping Agency's list of banned substances.

Supplements of the amino acids Ornithine, Arginine, and Lysine are marketed with the promise that they will stimulate the release of growth hormone and, in turn, enhance the growth of muscles. Large doses of these Amino Acids have been shown to stimulate the release of growth hormone. However, growth hormone levels in the blood of athletes taking these amino acids are no greater than levels typically resulting from exercise alone.

Also, supplements of these amino acids have not been found to cause greater increases in muscle mass and strength than those achieved through strength-training exercise alone.

Supplements to Enhance Performance in Short, Intense Activities

A number of supplements are marketed to athletes who seek to improve performance in sports that depend on quick bursts of intense activity. Supplements of β-hydroxy-β-methylbutyrate, known as HMB, claim to increase strength and muscle growth and improve muscle recovery; however, the outcome of research studies has been variable.

Overall, studies have found a small increase in strength in previously untrained men, but the effects in trained weightlifters are trivial, as is the effect of HMB on body composition.

Bicarbonate is a supplement that may enhance performance in high-intensity activities. Because bicarbonate acts as a buffer in the body, supplementing it is thought to neutralize acid and thus delay fatigue and allow improved performance.

Taking sodium bicarbonate, which is just baking soda from the kitchen cupboard, before exercise has been found to have a moderately positive effect on performance in sports, such as sprint cycling and sprint swimming, which entail intense exercise lasting only 1 to 7 minutes, as well as to enhance endurance in longer continuous and intermittent exercise, such as running and cycling.

However, just because baking soda is an ingredient in your cookies does not mean that it is risk free. Many people experience abdominal cramps and diarrhea after taking sodium bicarbonate, and other possible side effects have not been carefully researched.

One of the most popular ergogenic supplements is **Creatine**. This nitrogen-containing compound is found primarily in Muscle, where it is used to make Creatine Phosphate (Following Figure).

Higher levels of Creatine and Creatine Phosphate provide more quick Energy for short-term muscular activity. Creatine supplementation has been shown to increase muscle creatine phosphate levels and improve performance in high-intensity exercise lasting 30 seconds or less.

It is therefore beneficial for exercise that requires explosive bursts of energy, such as sprinting and weightlifting, but not for long-term endurance activities, such as marathons.

Athletes also take creatine supplements to increase muscle mass and strength. Creatine in combination with resistance training has been found to increase muscle strength and size more than resistance training alone.

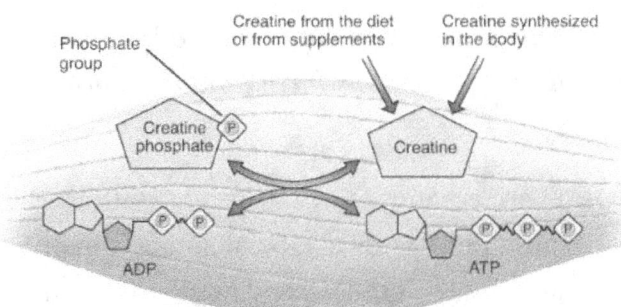

Creatine boosts or increases the production of Creatine Phosphate

Creatine can be synthesized in the Liver and Kidneys and is consumed in the diet in animal meat and milk. The *more* Creatine consumed, the greater the amount of Creatine stored in the Muscles. Increasing Creatine intake with supplement use has been shown to increase levels of Muscle Creatine and Creatine Phosphate, which is made from it.

During short bursts of intense activity, the Creatine Phosphate can transfer a Phosphate group to ADP, forming Creatine, and ATP that can be used for Muscle Contraction = Work.

Supplements to Enhance Endurance

Sprinters and weightlifters can benefit from increases in creatine phosphate levels, but endurance athletes are more concerned about running out of Glycogen.

Glycogen is spared when Fat is used as an energy source, allowing exercise to continue for a longer time before Glycogen is depleted and fatigue sets in.

Supplements that increase the amount of Fat or Oxygen available to the Muscle Cells are used to increase endurance.

Carnitine supplements are marketed as fat burners—substances that increase the utilization of fat during exercise. Carnitine is needed to transport Fatty Acids into the Mitochondria, where they are used to produce ATP by Aerobic Metabolism. Carnitine is ingested from the consumption of *Red Meats* and Dairy products, and it is also synthesized in the body.

Even when dietary carnitine is low, enough carnitine is made in the body to ensure efficient use of fatty acids. Carnitine supplements have not been shown to increase endurance.

Medium-chain triglycerides (MCT) are composed of fatty acids with medium-length carbon chains (8 to 10 carbons). These fatty acids can be absorbed directly into the blood without first being incorporated into Chylomicrons. They are therefore absorbed quickly, causing blood fatty acids levels to rise and thereby increasing the availability of fat as a fuel for exercise. ***Nevertheless, research has not found that supplementation with MCT increases endurance, spares glycogen, or enhances performance***.

Caffeine is a Stimulant found in Coffee, tea, soft drinks, and energy drinks. Consuming 3 to 6 mg of caffeine per kilogram of body weight, an amount equivalent to about 2.5 cups of percolated coffee, up to an hour before exercising as well as consuming smaller doses of caffeine during exercise (1 to 2 mg/kg) have been shown to improve endurance.

Caffeine *enhances* the release of Fatty Acids. When these Fatty Acids are used as a fuel source, less Glycogen is used, and the onset of Fatigue is delayed. *Athletes who are unaccustomed to caffeine respond better to it than do those who consume caffeine routinely*. Caffeine is also noted for its properties that improves concentration and enhances alertness, but in some athletes, it may impair performance by causing gastrointestinal upset or caffeine toxicity symptoms.

The popularity of energy drinks with names like Red Bull, Monster, and Full Throttle has soared over the past decade. They promise to keep you alert to study, work, drive, party all night, and perhaps excel at your next athletic competition.

The main ingredients in these drinks are Sugar and Caffeine. Glucose is an important fuel for exercise, and Caffeine is known to enhance endurance, so these drinks may seem like an ideal Ergogenic aid.

A traditional sports drink, like Gatorade, contains about 28 g of sugar in 16 oz; a typical energy drink provides twice this much (55 to 60 g, or about 14 teaspoons).

Since Carbohydrates fuels activity, it may seem that the additional sugar would provide energy for prolonged exercise. But more is not always better during activity.

The double load of sugar cannot be absorbed quickly, and unabsorbed sugar in the stomach can cause GI distress and also slow fluid absorption.

The caffeine content of energy drinks ranges from 50 to about 500 mg per can or bottle. Caffeine is an effective ergogenic aid that enhances endurance when consumed before or during exercise. *But too much caffeine, referred to as Caffeine Toxicity, causes nervousness, anxiety, restlessness, insomnia, gastrointestinal upset, tremors, increased blood pressure, and rapid heartbeat.*

A number of cases of caffeine-associated death, seizure, and cardiac arrest have occurred after consumption of energy drinks. Even if the caffeine in an energy drink increases endurance, depending on when it is consumed, it can affect timing and coordination and hurt overall performance.

How much caffeine is in your beverage?				
Beverage	Serving (fluid ounces)	Caffeine (mg)	Sugar (g)	Energy (Calories)
Coffee	8	100–200	0	0
Coca-Cola Classic	8	23	26	93
Mountain Dew	8	36	31	113
Monster	8	80	27	100
Jolt Cola	8	80	30	120
Arizona Caution Extreme Energy Shot	8	100	33	130
Red Bull	8	80	28	110
Rockstar	8	80	31	140
Full Throttle	8	80	28	110

Critical Thinking: Should you down an energy drink before your next competition? They do provide a caffeine boost, but is it so much caffeine that you risk dehydration, high blood pressure, and heart problems?

Energy drinks provide sugar to fuel activity, but will they upset your stomach? What about the herbal ingredients—do they offer a benefit you are looking for?

Caffeine is also a Diuretic; at the levels contained in these drinks, it may contribute to dehydration, particularly in first-time users. ***The FDA limits the amount of caffeine in soft drinks to 0.02% (about 71 mg in 12 oz), but energy drinks are considered dietary supplements, so the Caffeine content is not regulated.***

Energy drinks often also contain other ingredients that promise to improve performance, such as B vitamins, Taurine, Guarana, and Ginseng.

B Vitamins are needed to produce ATP, so they are marketed to enhance energy production from sugar. But unless you are deficient in these vitamins, drinking them in an energy drink will not enhance your ATP production.

Taurine is an amino acid that may reduce the amount of muscle damage and improve exercise performance and capacity, but not all research supports these claims.

Guarana is an herbal ingredient that contains caffeine as well as small amounts of the stimulants theobromine and theophylline. The extra caffeine from Guarana (not included in the caffeine listed for these beverages) may contribute to Caffeine Toxicity.

Ginseng is also claimed to have performance-enhancing effects, but these effects have not been demonstrated scientifically. In general, the amounts of these ingredients are too small to have much effect, and the safety of consuming them in combination with caffeine prior to or during exercise has yet to be established.

Other Supplements

In addition to the supplements discussed thus far, hundreds of other products are marketed to athletes. Most have no effect on performance.

For example, Brewer's Yeast is a source of B Vitamins and some Minerals but has not been found to have any Ergogenic properties. ***Likewise, there is no evidence to support claims that bee pollen or wheat germ oil enhances performance***.

Royal jelly is a substance that worker bees produce to help the queen bee grow larger and live longer, but it does not appear to enhance athletic capacity in humans.

Supplements of DNA and RNA are marketed to aid in tissue regeneration. DNA and RNA are needed to synthesize proteins, but they are not required in the diet, and supplements do not help replace damaged cells.

Herbal products are also marketed to athletes. Most have not been studied extensively for their ergogenic effects, so the only evidence of their benefits is anecdotal. Many can harm health as well as performance, so athletes should consider the risks before using these products.

*Chapter Fourteen....

Eating the Sun - Carbohydrates*

****

The Nature of Carbohydrate .. Basic Fuels: Sugars and Starch

Two forms of digestible **Carbohydrates** occur Naturally in plant foods: (1) Sugars and (2) Starch. Energy on planet Earth comes ultimately from the sun and its action on plants. Using their internal process of **Photosynthesis**, plants transform the sun's energy into the stored fuel of carbohydrate. Plants use carbon dioxide (CO_2) from the air and water from the soil—with the plant pigment Chlorophyll as a chemical catalyst—to manufacture these Natural Sugars and Starch. The carbs that plants store for their own energy needs become a source of fuel for us = Human Food.

 Because our bodies can rapidly break down Starch and Sugars, Carbs are often referred to as *Quick Energy Foods.* They are our primary source of energy.

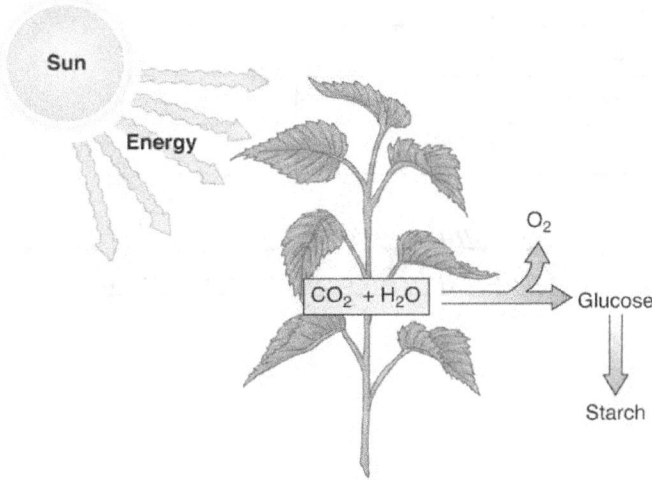

Functions of Carbohydrates

Energy

The primary function of these Starch and Sugars is to supply the necessary Energy to our Cells, especially our Brain Cells that **_depend_** on Glucose. When Carbs is lacking, Fats can be used as a temporary Energy source by most of our Organ systems; however, our Body Tissues require a constant supply of Glucose to function most efficiently.

Carbohydrates are the Foundation of The Human Energy System…..All Understanding has to BEGIN with Carbohydrates!

Body stores of Carbs are relatively small but still serve as an important Energy reserve. An adult man has about 300 to 350 grams of Carbohydrates stored in his Liver and Muscle in the form of Glycogen, and another 10 grams of Glucose circulates in his blood. Together, this Glycogen and Glucose will supply the Energy for only a half day of moderate activity. **_To meet the body's constant demand, Carbohydrate foods must be eaten regularly and at reasonably frequent intervals_**

	GLYCOGEN (g)	GLUCOSE (g)
Liver	72	
Muscles	245	
Extracellular fluids		10
Component totals	317	10
total storage	327	

The ONLY way to ensure this Constant and Consistent supply of Quality Life Energy manifested as Carbohydrates is to Grow and Harvest our own Food.

Classification of Carbohydrates

The term *Carbohydrate* comes from its Chemical nature. Carbohydrates contain the Essential Life Elements Carbon, Hydrogen, and Oxygen, with the hydrogen/oxygen ratio usually manifested as Water (CH_2O). Carbohydrates are classified according to the number of basic Sugar or Saccharide units that make up their structure.

PHYSIOLOGIC AND NUTRITIONAL SIGNIFICANCE OF MONOSACCHARIDES

MONOSACCHARIDE	SOURCE	SIGNIFICANCE
d-Glucose*	Fruit juices; hydrolysis of starch, cane sugar, maltose, and lactose	Form of sugar used by the body for fuel; found in blood and tissue fluids
d-Fructose	Fruit and fruit juices; honey; hydrolysis of sucrose from cane sugar	Converted to glucose in the liver and intestine to serve as body fuel
d-Galactose	Hydrolysis of lactose (milk sugar)	Converted to glucose in the liver to be used as body fuel; synthesized in the mammary gland to form lactose for milk; constituent of glycolipids and glycoproteins

Monosaccharides can exist in d or l forms depending on the position of the hydroxyl group on the right (d) or left (l) side of a specific carbon. Digestive enzymes are stereospecific and act only on d sugars.

The Monosaccharides and Disaccharides are referred to as *Simple Carbohydrates* because of their relatively small size and structure.

The polysaccharides, including Starch and certain Fibers, are called *Complex Carbohydrates* based on their larger size and more complicated structure.

Importance of Carbohydrates

The Complex Carb that is manifested in vegetables, legumes, and grains should be the major dietary source of Energy for us. When digested, Starch yields Glucose, the favorite energy source of Body Cells. ***Our Cells NEED Oxygen and Glucose!***

Fruit and dairy products supply Carbs in the form of naturally occurring Sugars (fruit contains Fructose, and milk contains Lactose). Vegetables, legumes, fruits, and grains (especially whole grains) supply other important nutrients, including vitamins, minerals, and fiber.

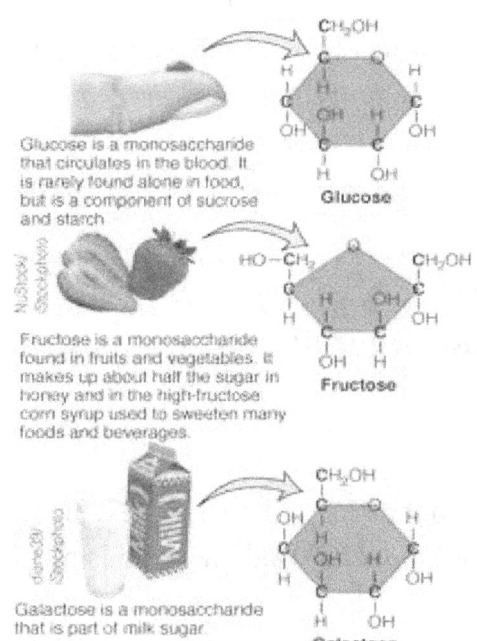

Glucose is a monosaccharide that circulates in the blood. It is rarely found alone in food, but is a component of sucrose and starch

Glucose

Fructose is a monosaccharide found in fruits and vegetables. It makes up about half the sugar in honey and in the high-fructose corn syrup used to sweeten many foods and beverages.

Fructose

Galactose is a monosaccharide that is part of milk sugar.

Galactose

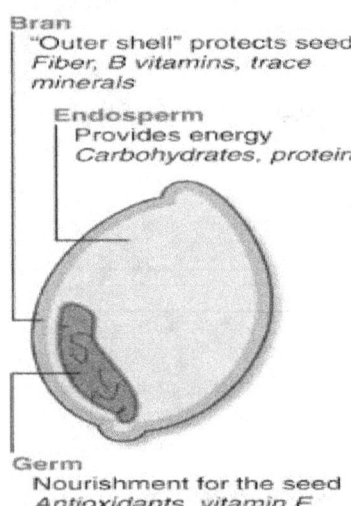

Whole grain kernel

Bran
"Outer shell" protects seed
*Fiber, B vitamins, trace
minerals*

Endosperm
Provides energy
Carbohydrates, protein

Germ
Nourishment for the seed
*Antioxidants, vitamin E,
B vitamins*

Dairy products are good sources of calcium, magnesium, and protein. Currently, major food sources of starch in the American diet are refined grains, such as white bread and ready-to-eat cereals, white potatoes, pasta, and rice, which are often highly processed and limited in micronutrients.

Whole grains include the bran covering of the grain kernel when compared with refined grains from which the bran has been removed. Refined grains are enriched with several B vitamins, iron, and folate but provide less fiber and other trace minerals. Carbohydrate foods high in added sugar supply kcalories but little else. Based on the connection between added sugar and cardiovascular risk factors, including obesity, the American Heart Association recommends a prudent intake not to exceed 100 kcal per day for women and 150 kcal for men.

Nutrients in the bran and germ of whole grains are lost when grains are refined and the bran and germ are discarded.

Current laws require that processed grains be enriched with thiamin, riboflavin, niacin, iron, and folate; however, other important nutrients such as zinc and vitamin E, also lost in processing, are not replaced. This can only be done through artificial means, which alters the state of the food-like product.

YOU ARE WHAT YOU EAT…..Eating an artificially modified or fortified food-like item releases artificial ENERGY….which causes a disruption in the Natural Energy that gives us LIFE!

Special Functions

As the Foundation of the Human Energy System, Carbohydrates have other specialized roles in our overall Body Metabolism.

Glycogen—Carbohydrate Storage

Liver and muscle glycogen are in constant interchange with the body's overall energy system. These energy reserves protect cells, especially brain cells, from depressed metabolic function and injury and support urgent muscle responses.

Protein-Sparing Action

Carbohydrates help regulate protein metabolism. An adequate supply of carbohydrate to satisfy ongoing energy demands prevents the channeling of protein for energy. This protein-sparing action of carbohydrate allows protein to be reserved for tissue building and repair.

Antiketogenic Effect

Carbohydrates influence fat metabolism. The supply of carbohydrate determines how much fat must be broken down to meet energy needs, thereby controlling the formation of *ketones*. Ketones are intermediate products of fat metabolism that normally are produced in very small amounts. However, when carbohydrate is inadequate to meet cell energy needs, as in starvation or uncontrolled diabetes or very low-carbohydrate diets, fat is oxidized at extreme rates. Sufficient amounts of dietary carbohydrates prevent any damaging excess of ketones.

Heart Action

Heart action is a life-sustaining muscle activity. Although fatty acids are the preferred fuel for the heart, the glycogen stored in cardiac muscle is an important emergency source of contractile energy.

Central Nervous System

The brain and central nervous system (CNS) depend on carbohydrate for energy but have very low carbohydrate reserves—enough to last only 10 to 15 minutes. This makes them especially dependent on a minute-to-minute supply of glucose from the blood.

Sustained *hypoglycemic* shock causes irreversible brain damage. Providing an adequate morning supply of glucose for brain function may help to explain why individuals who eat breakfast do better in school than those who skip breakfast.[19] Glucose increases the synthesis of acetylcholine, a neurotransmitter that acts on areas of the brain responsible for memory and cognitive function

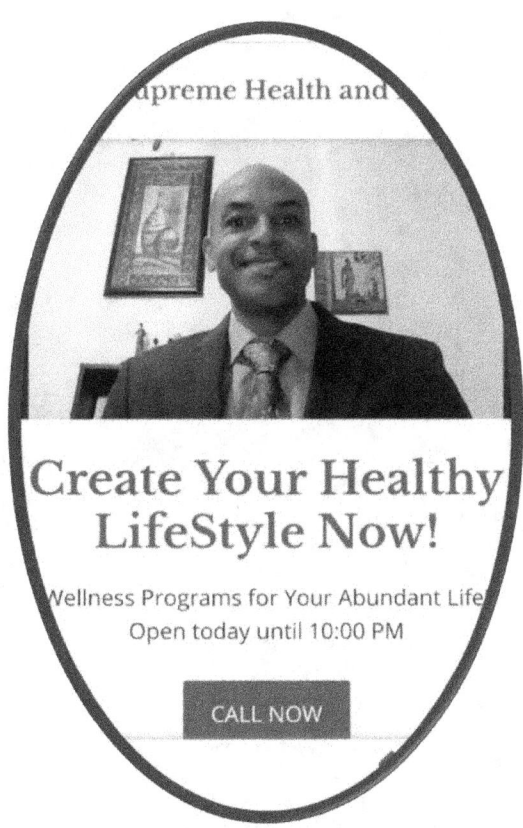

Conclusion

Peace & Blessings!

I Sincerely and very Humbly offer my THANK YOU for reading my small labor of Love. It was/is my intentions to offer a New Health Paradigm whenever we are Proactive and have a new Understanding of Health and Healing. Our Bodies are WONDERFUL Vehicles, Perfectly Designed by Our CREATOR to successfully carry us through Time, able to Build and Enjoy all the Awesome Bounties of Life.

With this book, I wanted to present the best scientific and medical research and data available so that we can make the best possible Energy or food choices as possible.

It is only through our **lack** of knowledge of Self- HOW we function, and WHAT Human Energy is that causes us to suffer dis-eases and pre-mature death

We are created to literally Live as long as we want to. A majority of the dis-eases that causes pre-mature death are food-borne or related. The main cause = Eating Other-than HUMAN food!

We are WHAT we Eat and we die or LIVE accordingly.....But the choice is YOURS!

HOW long do you want to LIVE?

Considering the vast amount of Genetically Altered or Modified foods that are the majority of commercial food-like items are made of, it is Time.....RIGHT NOW ...for us to GROW OUR OWN FOOD...!!!!

Eating according to our Anatomical Structure and Functions is the foundation for Successfully Building Supreme Health and Fitness.

Eating the foods that The Creator designed for us allows us to Manifest the Highest Qualities of Humanity = The Direct Express Image & Likeness of The CREATOR!

Do YOU want to Enjoy ABUNDANT LIFE?

IF YOU DON'T HAVE A LIFE GARDEN ALREADY ESTABLISHED......PLEASE PUT THIS BOOK DOWN AND GO START ONE!!!!

Let Us be Found Eating To LIVE!

Peace!

*Charts * Figures * Graphs*

****

Body Mass Index: Obesity Values

BMI	36	37	38	39	40	41	42	43	44	45	46	47	48	49	50	51	52	53	54

HEIGHT (INCHES)   BODY WEIGHT (POUNDS)

Height	36	37	38	39	40	41	42	43	44	45	46	47	48	49	50	51	52	53	54
58	172	177	181	186	191	196	201	205	210	215	220	224	229	234	239	244	248	253	258
59	178	183	188	193	198	203	208	212	217	222	227	232	237	242	247	252	257	262	267
60	184	189	194	199	204	209	215	220	225	230	235	240	245	250	255	261	266	271	276
61	190	195	201	206	211	217	222	227	232	238	243	248	254	259	264	269	275	280	285
62	196	202	207	213	218	224	229	235	240	246	251	256	262	267	273	278	284	289	295
63	203	208	214	220	225	231	237	242	248	254	259	265	270	278	282	287	293	299	304
64	209	215	221	227	232	238	244	250	256	262	267	273	279	285	291	296	302	308	314
65	216	222	228	234	240	246	252	258	264	270	276	282	288	294	300	306	312	318	324
66	223	229	235	241	247	253	260	266	272	278	284	291	297	303	309	315	322	328	334
67	230	236	242	249	255	261	268	274	280	287	293	299	306	312	319	325	331	338	344
68	236	243	249	256	262	269	276	282	289	295	302	308	315	322	328	335	341	348	354
69	243	250	257	263	270	277	284	291	297	304	311	318	324	331	338	345	351	358	365
70	250	257	264	271	278	285	292	299	306	313	320	327	334	341	348	355	362	369	376
71	257	265	272	279	286	293	301	308	315	322	329	338	343	351	358	365	372	379	386
72	265	272	279	287	294	302	309	316	324	331	338	346	353	361	368	375	383	390	397
73	272	280	288	295	302	310	318	325	333	340	348	355	363	371	378	386	393	401	408
74	280	287	295	303	311	319	326	334	342	350	358	365	373	381	389	396	404	412	420
75	287	295	303	311	319	327	335	343	351	359	367	375	383	391	399	407	415	423	431
76	295	304	312	320	328	336	344	353	361	369	377	385	394	402	410	418	426	435	443

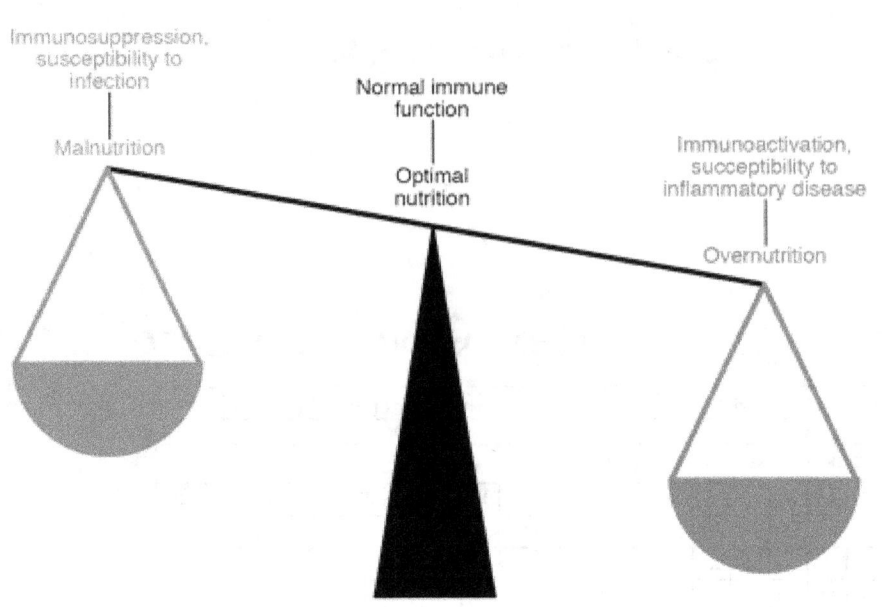

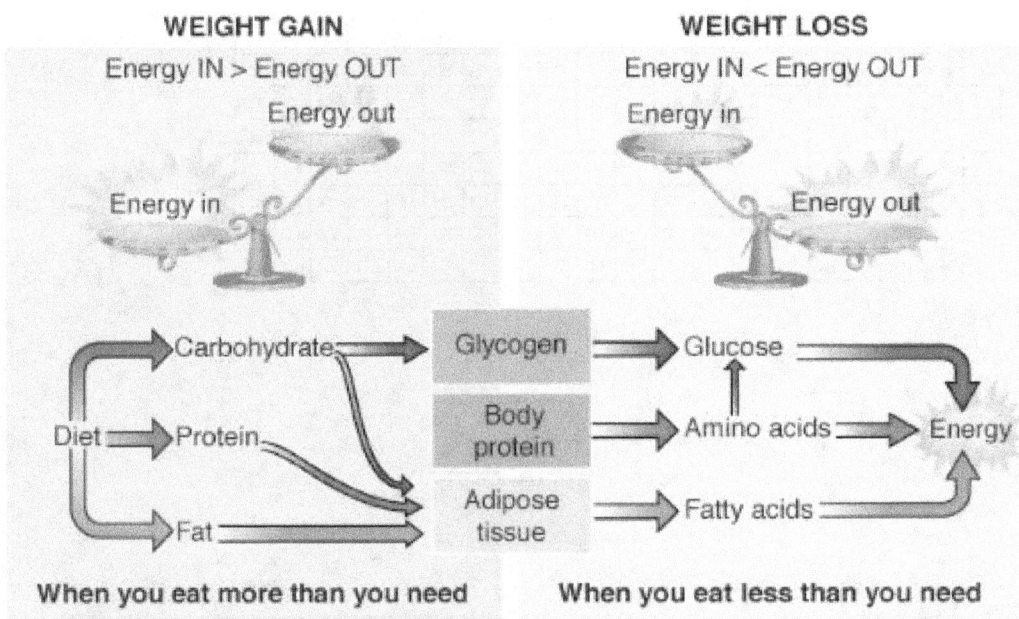

Energy transformations in the human body are accompanied with continuous production of heat

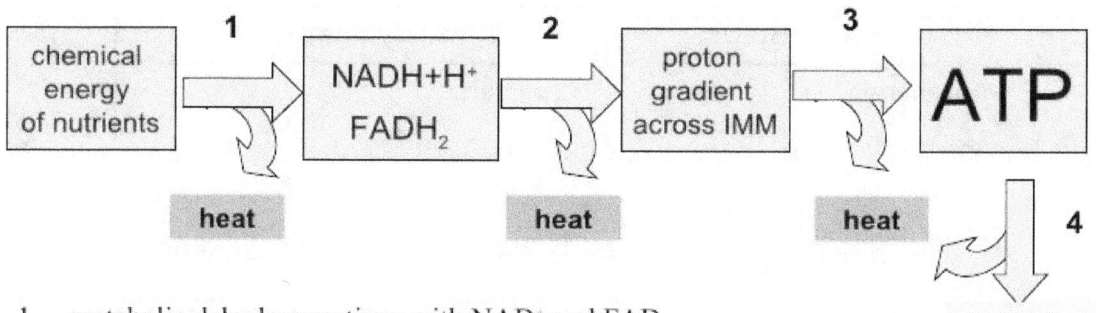

1 ... metabolic dehydrogenations with NAD^+ and FAD

2 ... respiratory chain (oxidation of reduced cofactors + reduction of O_2 to H_2O)

3 ... oxidative phosphorylation, IMM inner mitochondrial membrane

4 ... transformation of chemical energy of ATP into work + some heat

 ... high energy systems   4

TABLE 2.1   Estimated Energy Stores in Humans

Energy source	Storage site	Approximate energy (kcal)
ATP/CP*	Various tissues	5
Carbohydrate	Blood glucose	80
	Liver glycogen	400
	Muscle glycogen	1,500
Fat	Serum free fatty acids	7
	Serum triglycerides	75
	Muscle triglycerides	2,500
	Adipose tissue	80,000+
Protein	Muscle protein	30,000

*ATP/CP = adenosine triphosphate/creatine phosphate

	Sympathetic	Parasympathetic
Synonym	Adrenergic	Cholinergic
Preganglionic fiber	Short	Long
Neurohumoral agent*	Acetylcholine	Acetylcholine
Ganglion location	Paravertebral	End organ
Postganglionic fiber	Long	Short
Neurohumoral agent*	Norepinephrine	Acetylcholine
Extraautonomic sites	Adrenal medulla	Neuromuscular junction
Evolutionary role	Fight-flight/defense-alarm	Relaxation response, vegetative functions
Activators	Multiple	Specific
Blockers	Diffuse, nonspecific	Selective, cholinesterase
Degradative enzymes	Monoamine oxidase, methyltransferase	

References

****

1. Popkin, BM. What can public health nutritionists do to curb the epidemic of nutrition-related noncommunicable disease? *Nutr Rev*. 2009; 67(Suppl 1):S79.

2. Centers for Disease Control and Prevention, *Overweight and obesity. Data and statistics. Adult obesity facts*. Centers for Disease Control and Prevention, Atlanta, Ga., 2012. at. http://www.cdc.gov/obesity/data/adult.html [Accessed on September 8, 2013].

3. Flegal, KM, Carroll, MD, Kit, BK, et al. Prevalence of obesity and trends in the distribution of body mass index among US adults, 1999-2012. *JAMA*. 2012; 307(5):491.

4. Ogden, CL, Carroll, MD, Kit, BK, et al. Prevalence of obesity and trends in body mass index among US children and adolescents, 1999-2010. *JAMA*. 2012; 307(5):483.

5. Centers for Disease Control and Prevention, *Diabetes data and trends. Number (in millions) of civilian, noninstitutionalized persons with diagnosed diabetes, United States, 1980-2011*. National Center for Chronic Disease Prevention and Health Promotion, Centers for Disease Control and Prevention, Division of Diabetes Translation, Atlanta, Ga., 2011. at. http://www.cdc.gov/diabetes/statistics/prev/national/figpersons.htm [Accessed on January 25, 2013].

6. Centers for Disease Control and Prevention, *National diabetes fact sheet: national estimates and general information on diabetes and prediabetes in the United States, 2011*. U.S. Department of Health and Human Services, Centers for Disease Control and Prevention, Atlanta, Ga., 2011. at. http://www.cdc.gov/diabetes/pubs/pdf/ndfs_2011.pdf [Accessed on August 19, 2013].

7. Chaput, JP, Doucet, E, Tremblay, A. Obesity: a disease or a biological adaptation? An update. *Obes Rev*. 2012; 13:681.

8. Frank, LD, Saelens, BE, Chapman, J, et al. Objective assessment of obesogenic environments in youth. Geographic information system methods and spatial findings from the Neighborhood Impact on Kids Study. *Am J Prev Med*. 2012; 42(5):e47.

9. Ledikwe, JH, Ello-Martin, JA, Rolls, BJ. Portion sizes and the obesity epidemic. *J Nutr*. 2005; 135:905.

10. Piernas, C, Popkin, BM. Food portion patterns and trends among U.S children and the relationship to total eating occasion size, 1977-2006. *J Nutr*. 2011; 141:1159.

11. Federal Interagency Forum on Aging-Related Statistics. *Older Americans 2012: Key indicators of well-being*. Washington, D.C.: U.S. Government Printing Office; 2012.

12. Henry J Kaiser Family Foundation, *Health Care Costs: A Primer. Key Information on Health Care Costs and Their Impact, Publ 7670-03* Menlo Park, Calif., 2012. at. http://kaiserfamilyfoundation.files.wordpress.com/2013/01/7670-03.pdf [Accessed on January 25, 2013].

13. United States Census Bureau, *Statistical Abstract of the United States*, ed 131, 2012. Washington, D.C.; at. http://www.census.gov/compendia/statab/ [Accessed on August 19, 2013].

14. Goody, CM, Drago, L. *Cultural Food Practices, American Dietetic Association (now the Academy of Nutrition and Dietetics)*. Chicago, Ill.: Diabetes Care and Education Dietetic Practice Group; 2010.

15. United States Bureau of Census, *Selected social characteristics in the United States, 2011 American Community Survey 1-year estimates, American FactFinder, DP02*. U.S. Department of Commerce, Washington, D.C., 2011. at. http://factfinder2.census.gov/faces/tableservices/jsf/pages/productview.xhtml?pid=ACS_11_1YR_DP02&prodType=table [Accessed on January 25, 2013].

16. American Dietetic Association. Position of the American Dietetic Association: functional foods. *J Am Diet Assoc*. 2009; 109:735.

17. Djousse, L, Hopkins, PN, North, KE, et al. Chocolate consumption is inversely associated with prevalent coronary 23heart disease: The National Heart, Lung, and Blood Institute Family Heart Study. *Clin Nutr*. 2011; 30:182.

Further Reading and Resources

****

Readings

Academy of Nutrition and Dietetics. Position of the Academy of Nutrition and Dietetics: total diet approach to healthy eating. *J Acad Nutr Diet*. 2013; 113:307.

[This review helps us understand the importance of the overall food pattern, not just one day or one meal.]

Klurfeld, DM. What do government agencies consider in the debate over added sugars? *Adv Nutr*. 2013; 4(2):257.

[Dr. Klurfeld reviews the trends in added sugar intake and the health implications for the American public.]

25 Reilly, PR, DeBusk, RM. Ethical and legal issues in nutritional genomics. *J Am Diet Assoc*. 2008; 108:36.

[When it becomes possible to customize nutrition intervention based on an individual's genetic code, there are various issues that will need to be considered.]

Slavin, J. Dietary Guidelines. Are we on the right path? *Nutr Today*. 2012; 47(5):245.

[This nutrition expert raises questions about the 2010 Dietary Guidelines and provides suggestions for change when the 2015 Guidelines are developed.]

U.S. Department of Agriculture, Center for Nutrition Policy and Promotion, *An evidence-based approach to reviewing the science on nutrition and health, Nutrition Insight 38*. U.S. Government Printing Office, Alexandria, Va., 2008. from. http://www.cnpp.usda.gov/Publications/NutritionInsights/Insight38.pdf [Retrieved on August 19, 2013].

[This publication provides a helpful summary on why we need to apply an evidence-based approach to our practice and gives an example of the process.]

U.S. Department of Agriculture, Center for Nutrition Policy and Promotion, *The Food Environment, Eating Out, and Body Weight: A Review of the Evidence, Nutrition Insight 49*. U.S. Government Printing Office, Alexandria, Va., 2012. from. http://www.cnpp.usda.gov/Publications/NutritionInsights/Insight49.pdf [Retrieved on August 19, 2013].

[This review cites evidence from the Nutrition Evidence Library (NEL) linking frequency of meals away from home and risk of overweight, and helps us understand why this occurs.]

Wellman, NS, Borra, ST, Schleman, JC, et al. Trends in news media reporting of food and health issues. *Nutr Today*. 2011; 46(3):123. [May-June].

[These authors help us understand how and why nutrition and health misinformation gets publicized and how we as health professionals can address this.]

Websites of Interest

• U.S. Department of Agriculture: Nutrition Evidence Library, 2013. This website provided the scientific evidence reviewed by the 2010 Dietary Guidelines Advisory Committee in preparation of their report. http://www.cnpp.usda.gov/NEL.htm.

• U.S. Department of Health and Human Services, 2008. *Physical Activity Guidelines for Americans*. This Web site presents science-based physical activity guidelines for both youth and adults along with educational materials for health professionals and consumers. http://www.health.gov/paguidelines/guidelines/default.aspx.

• U.S. Department of Agriculture, Food Surveys Research Group: *What We Eat in America: Data from the National Health and Nutrition Examination Survey*. This site describes the food and nutrient intakes of Americans according to age, sex, race, ethnicity, and economic status. www.ars.usda.gov/Services/docs.htm?docid=15044.

• U.S. Department of Health and Human Services, National Heart, Lung and Blood Institute: *Keep an Eye on Portion Distortion*. This site describes portion sizes and how they have changed over the years. http://hp2010.nhlbihin.net/portion/keep.htm.

• U.S. Department of Agriculture, Center for Nutrition Policy and Promotion. The MyPlate (ChooseMyPlate.gov) website offers materials for health professionals and practical tips for consumers to use in meal planning; www.ChooseMyPlate.gov.

• Nestle Nutrition, Clinical Resources and Tools. This site provides tools and resources to help identify, assess, and select appropriate products to address the nutrition challenges of patients: www.nestle-nutrition.com/Clinical_Resources/Default.aspx.

• U.S. Department of Agriculture, Food and Nutrition Information Center, Dietary Analysis and Intake Calculators. This site, hosted by the Food and Nutrition Information Center (FNIC) at the National Agricultural Library (NAL), provides links to numerous diet-analysis tools: http://fnic.nal.usda.gov/dietary-guidance/interactive-tools

Sean Ali

Understanding Carbohydrates: LIFE Energy, Fiber, Sugar and Starch! (Science Of LIFE Series)

ISBN-13: 978-1520559988, **ISBN-10:** 1520559984

#1 New Release in Fiber

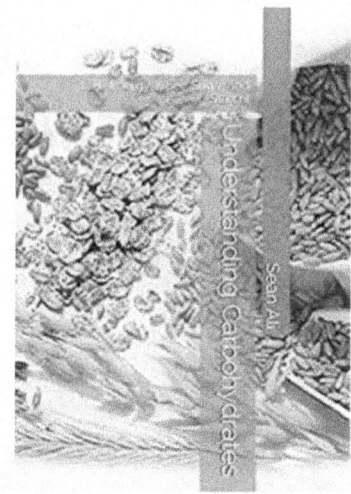

www.ingramcontent.com/pod-product-compliance
Lightning Source LLC
Chambersburg PA
CBHW081111180526
45170CB00008B/2804